DIETING FOR DECADES

A Sustainable Approach Built to Last a Lifetime

by Henry Barry and Mark Barry

With illustrations by Missy Quick

CONTENTS

COPYRIGHT

◆ ◆ ◆

CHAPTER 1: INTRODUCTION

◆ ◆ ◆

The best diet is not the one that makes you lose weight the fastest - it is the one that gets you to your goal and keeps you there for as much of your life as possible.

Most diet books are written by people who have dedicated every moment of their professional lives to researching and perfecting their nutrition. These people earn their livelihoods by studying dieting and implementing healthy habits for themselves. Their entire careers are designed to optimize their diets.

This is part of the problem: most people's careers are not related to their diets. In fact, most careers often work against nutritional progress. For most of us, learning about dieting is an extracurricular activity that gets pushed in-between dozens of other important things we have to take care of when we're not working.

Reading a diet book by a person whose entire life is built for their ease of dieting is like learning how to wash your car from someone who is a full-time Ferrari-detailer. They may give you some great detailing tips, but you will quickly be overwhelmed when they explain to you that a good wash and wax takes eight hours and $100 of equipment. Meanwhile, you have a Honda Accord, and are just trying to get the bird crap off the hood. You don't need an exquisite detailing befitting an Italian sports car. You just need your car to look clean. The sophistication is not only wasted, it can be so complicated that it turns you off from actually improving your diet in the first place.

Similarly, in dieting, incredible books have been written by some of the world's smartest PhD's. They have cutting-edge recipes and practices, but the wheels fall off quickly when you realize that your grocery bill is about to triple, your time spent cooking will quadruple, and you will be eating nothing but asparagus and organic lentils for the rest of your life. This is overkill for most people. It you are like many of us, you just need to cut out some of the bad habits and foods from your diet and need a push to get there, not the world-class, perfect human diet.

To address the Ferrari-detailer paradox, we bring you the opposite: a book written by someone with no formal background in dietary science and a boatload of other commitments that ensure I have very limited time and resources to focus on my eating. My life is the opposite of the laboratory conditions that many world-class diet books assume.

You may be disappointed, because this sounds like instead of getting the Ferrari, you are getting the Accord. You are. That is by design. Extending the driving metaphor, you have only recently started driving, and the power and intricacy of the Ferrari would be overwhelming. In dieting terms, this means that you are not ready to eat only asparagus and lentils. Honestly, you probably wouldn't really enjoy the Ferrari if you had it, because having it means you would never get to deviate from Dr. PhD's diet.

Dr. PhD's diet isn't real life, it is becoming Ivan Drago from Rocky IV: a machine-like monster whose entire existence is centered around perfect diet and exercise. We'll start with small steps, make some progress with the Accord, and once we do that, see if we even need to get more granular. If so, there are dozens of more detailed books you can dig into. You may continue to seek knowledge and achieve Ferrari-level sophistication with your diet, but you may also decide you don't need that. You may get fit and have abs and call it a day. But starting with the most complex, difficult solution will increase your chances of failing.

I've enlisted my father, Mark Barry, to provide his input as well, because a diet book written by a 26 year old just isn't applicable to everyone. It can be written off as the luck of a youthful metabolism. But add in the experience of a 57 year-old and you suddenly have concepts that cover most of a lifetime.

My father and I have watched each other fluctuate weight and have adventured through diets both normal and strange (Dad, you'll never live down the bagged tuna on Triscuits lunch!). Over the years, we've spent a lot of time talking through how the body changes and how to adapt. This book represents the culmination of all our conversations and experiments. My father's perspective is denoted by the words in italics, but since we generally agree philosophically, my words represent him as well unless otherwise noted.

We aren't dietitians. We are just regular people who have managed to get and stay healthy, leading normal lives with stressful jobs. We travel, we have business dinners, parties, and eat out with our friends. We want to live our lives and not work harder than we have to on dieting. Our mission has been to find a system that works to achieve our dieting goals, stack the cards in our favor so that it continues to work, and then cruise. We believe that there is more to life than dieting, and we seek the path of maximum efficiency, not the path of perfection, to get us to our goals.

This attitude is the product of today's business world. Mark has had a long and successful career running and improving multi-national companies, using a laser-like focus on what is important and disregarding everything else. Similarly, through my time working in the asset management industry and through a financial professional designation program (the Chartered Financial Analyst curriculum), I've come to understand the harsh reality of behavioral biases. Most people act irrationally and take the path of least resistance, becoming slaves to the easy option.

In my day job, this manifests itself most clearly through people's retirement accounts. For many Americans, the assets in their 401(k) account will fund a large portion of their lifestyle in retirement. Yet despite this, most employees spend very little time paying attention to their 401(k). Do you? When was the last time you checked your 401(k)? Do you monitor it regularly? How much do you contribute? Have you increased that since you started working? Do you even have one set up?

If you are early in your career and are paying attention to your 401(k), good for you. You are relatively rare. Most people stay in whatever 401(k) investment option they are defaulted into. The majority of people don't understand investments, and they don't remember to check their 401(k) balances frequently. As a response to this, most companies automatically enroll employees into diversified target date funds that do all the rebalancing for the employees. Many companies set an automatic contribution amount for new employees, and often set automatic escalation up so that every year, employees are defaulted into contributing a little bit more.

This system has worked remarkably well to improve people's retirement outcomes because it has made success the default option. By making the default option one that works, and allowing people to opt-out if they want something different, companies have capitalized on people's inherent laziness to help them. This is exactly what we plan to do with your diet.

While the benefits departments of many large companies have started to take advantage of people's propensity to do very little, many diets have not yet caught on. In fact, many take the opposite approach, and add significant amounts of additional work and complexity. Our goal is to throw that on its head and build a system that is easier and lasts longer.

If you want a diet to work for your whole life, you have to make it incredibly easy for yourself to succeed. Not just easier, but as easy as you possibly can. Knowledge alone won't do it for you: you need easy actions that don't require herculean effort. That is where we come in. We're here to show you little ways that you can make big progress without ruining your life or being a slave to tough decisions.

Why Write This?

"The mass of men lead lives of quiet desperation."

While Henry David Thoreau wasn't talking about the futility of weight loss when he wrote this in the 1800s, it describes most people's fitness situation. Whatever people are trying to do, it isn't working. There are plenty of great dieting books out there, but clearly people either aren't reading them, or the knowledge in them isn't sticking, because seventy percent of Americans are overweight and thirty-seven percent are obese[1].

Just think about that for a second. If you put 100 random Americans in a room, only 30 would not be overweight. More people would be obese than would be skinny. I'll save you the rant about the damage this is causing to our healthcare system and leave you with the question: how many people, as kids, decide they want to be fat when they grow up?

Maybe some people do want to be heavy for whatever reason, but it likely isn't 70% of the population. If everyone was happy with their weight, the health and fitness industry would not be one of the fastest-growing industries, worth billions of dollars.

A more interesting question is how the non-overweight Americans feel. Are they happy? How many are effortlessly skinny, and how many feel like it takes a mountain of work just to stay in place and not fall into the 70%? How many of these 30% will remain at a healthy weight throughout their lifetimes, and how many will slowly gain weight over the years until they join the majority?

Common across almost everyone in the United States is either an inability to maintain a healthy weight, or a huge amount of effort to do so. We are doing something wrong.

Even more frustrating is that for many people, it seems like they are doing everything right, but they still aren't having the results they would expect. Some people are running, biking, and eating nothing but lettuce, but still don't have six pack abs.

Some of us just can't seem to muster up the willpower to hold ourselves back from eating things we know we shouldn't, while others effortlessly glide past tempting foods.

Many people are missing part of the puzzle.

Not all of it. Most people do a few things right, but if they were doing everything right, they would be out there with the bodies they want, doing something way more fun than reading books like this.

The problem is that the world has changed, but nutritional education and behavioral best practices have not caught up. A century ago, people could just not think about their diets and they would, for the most part, stay skinny. Portion sizes were small. Most people worked manual labor or outdoor jobs. Smart phones, the internet, and video games didn't exist, so people had to entertain themselves with more calorie-intensive activities. Many processed foods had not yet even been invented. Few people had to put forth any effort to be skinny.

Today it is the opposite: if you don't pay attention, you will likely be overweight. It isn't your fault and does not mean you are lazy. It just means you are a product of your environment, and today's environment is very fattening. If you want to change your body composition, or make your dieting easier, behavioral change is helpful, but changes to your environment may be more important to make long-term progress.

This book will help you understand just how much of an uphill battle this can be, and will equip you to succeed as quickly as possible. I'm going to make this as to-the-point and actionable as I can because life is too short to read diet books.

Before we get into things, I need something from you. I need you to take everything you think you know, and press pause. Open up and know that this isn't going to be like every other diet book you've read before.

You are likely frustrated because you have tried before, and failed. You've done what people recommended, and it didn't work. You feel like something is wrong with you - that you're different. Here's the thing: in some ways, you are. There are certain habits and foods that your body will respond well to. Yet the overarching principles remain the same for everyone. We are going to help you find the habits and foods that work for you while also understanding the broad principles that apply to everyone.

It doesn't matter what someone else said would work for you, or what you think you are supposed to do. All that matters is that you find things that give you the results you want. These may be a lot easier than you'd think, or a lot harder. It doesn't matter. Stop worrying about your diet conflicting with other diets or other practices that other people do. If you find the one that works for you, you win. End of story. So just pause everything you think is right and change your focus to finding what your body responds to.

To be clear, dieting is about results, not effort. Nobody gets an "A" for effort in dieting. If you're focusing on the wrong things, trying harder doesn't win you any awards. So put away your tough guy (or girl) attitude and be ok with the fact that you may not always be straining to the limits of your willpower. Sometimes you will, but we are trying to create a framework that lasts for decades, not a six week sprint. You will get there in the long run, but if you try to sprint the whole way there you may burn out and give up.

The Octopus

Part of the reason so many people fail when dieting is that they focus on only a few factors, and changing your body composition requires change in a lot of different dimensions.

Imagine that there's a monster that is constantly trying to attach itself to you and slowly leach away your happiness. It has two tentacles that you fight off, but even pushing those away usually isn't enough to stop it from overpowering you, and you don't understand why.

Once it attaches itself to you and starts sucking away at your well-being, it is very tough to get off. The longer it stays attached to you, the harder it is to remove. You spend all of your time thinking of new ways to outmaneuver and overpower its two tentacles, and you often win against those, but somehow, as if by magic, it still manages to attach itself to you.

One day, you see clearly and realize that the monster doesn't have two tentacles - it has eight. You had never paid any attention to the other six, which explains why even when you'd bested the original two, the other six would wrap themselves around you and attach the octopus to you. By missing all eight, you were doomed to fail in all but the most ideal conditions.

This is a lot like dieting. Most people focus with fanatical intensity on a few variables - eating more lettuce and exercising more - and totally ignore the rest of the picture. They may be crushing those two goals, but miss the bigger picture of other factors that matter for their health. They may be eating a lot of lettuce and exercising, but that goes out the window any time they get stressed or travel. Their system only addresses some variables, and isn't built to adapt to changing situations.

The two main tentacles, diet and exercise, are important, and most people focus on them for good reason. To be fair, most people are able to dial those in for short periods of time. However, the way most people focus on them is to come at the octopus with a sword and chop them off at the end of one or two tentacles. That works - for a few weeks. But it doesn't address the bigger problem: that there is an octopus with six tentacles left trying to get them! The octopus still chases them, and often clings on with the other six tentacles, and before they know it, the octopus is fully attached again. Then the two tentacles grow back and the whole scene repeats.

The other six tentacles represent everything else in your life that complicates you getting to your goals. Friends, family, and co-workers that want you to eat unhealthy foods. Stress from work that can be mitigated with some sweets. Sleep deprivation caused by business trips, family, or whatever other excuse you have. While these other tentacles are unique to each person, understanding them and finding ways to work around them them is key to your success. Many times, they are hard to see and keep track of, because they are constantly changing, and may even seem inconsequential. Yet if you want to beat the octopus, you have to be aware of and fight all eight of the tentacles.

This is more than just a onetime fight. Our goal is to show you a way to keep the octopus away for good. To put it in a cage out of reach so it won't constantly attack you. You can never kill the octopus, but you can weaken it and keep it at a safe distance so you rarely have to deal with it. The longer you keep it away from you, the weaker it gets, and the easier it is to keep away. Its tentacles will always reach out to you if you get too close, and it will always try to attach itself to you, and it sometimes may succeed, but we will give you the tools to keep it under control. It will best you sometimes, because life happens, but you will know how to fight it and put it back into its cage.

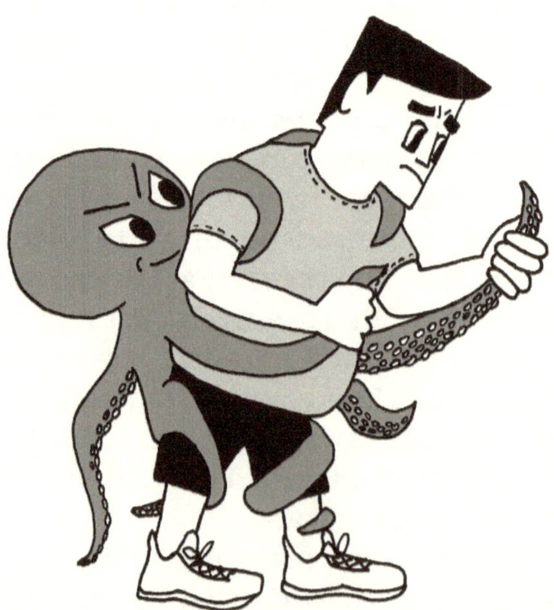

Mark here - I really like the Octopus analogy, but I do feel the need to defend Octopi. They are beautiful, intelligent, and otherworldly creatures, not monsters. That said, the tentacles are quite tasty when grilled!

This will be an uphill battle. If you aren't careful, you might be right back where you started. Most of America is overweight, because if you make the default decisions and do what most people do, you end up too heavy. The way to win is changing your default decisions and making them effortless.

Even if you can do that, the deck is stacked against you. First, your body is generally happy being heavier, and often would rather gain weight than lose it. We have evolution to thank: this is an adaptation that increases your odds of survival by leading you to have extra fat reserves. Second, there are entire industries that make money off of you being overweight and have an incentive for you to remain that way.

The supplement and fitness industry, while overall likely a good thing, has a perverse conflict of interest in seeing your success. Here's the thing: if everyone actually achieved the bodies they wanted, what would these companies have to sell? There are a lot of vested interests that have a stake in you staying out of shape. So it is in their best interest for you to make some progress with their products, but be entirely dependent on them. While some of the products offered work, a lot either simply don't, or only work for a short period of time.

Similarly, the food industry does not care about your fitness. They may offer healthier options to cater to what customers want, but their goal is profit first, and much of that profit comes from cheap, processed ingredients with high margins. If you stopped buying fast food and snack foods, a lot of companies would lose a lot of money. They are bombarding us with advertising and scientifically-designed snacks that are created to maximize tastiness because their financial livelihoods depend on it.

With these obstacles, and the other individual ones you may have in your path, you need to arm yourself with every advantage you can.

The key is not fighting harder, it is having a strategy. More willpower may bring strong short-term results, but if all you have is willpower without strategy, your entire life will be a high-intensity struggle with constant ups and downs. Everything will be harder than it needs to be. A long-term strategy will let you coast with a lot less total effort. Sometimes you will need to apply yourself 100%, but you will have more time to put your diet on autopilot and simply enjoy your life.

Building a System

We are going to focus on finding ways that you are more likely to stick to healthy eating. To find solutions where you don't have to ostracize yourself socially. To create work-arounds for tasty things that aren't as bad for you. The focus will be on simple rules that keep you on the right track, and building a skill-set to make your own food so you aren't reliant on others to give you the nutrition you need, and don't have to pay for their expertise.

I will aim to make this as sustainable as possible and will hold the overarching assumption that you are a normal person that has a normal amount of willpower. You have all sorts of stressful things going on in your life, and you want to save your willpower for harder things than food. Your job and personal life test your resolve plenty, so don't waste any of it having to fight uphill dieting battles. You will still get to lead a normal life, but you'll do everything smarter. You will optimize and get the most enjoyment you possibly can while still making good decisions that lead you towards your goal.

This is the difference between doing a magazine diet: something with arbitrary and often difficult food restrictions and meal requirements that usually lasts somewhere between 6 and 12 weeks, and doing a lifelong diet: something you can follow for the rest of your life. Since you're often fighting your body and the people around you in your quest to get and stay fit, this truly is an uphill battle on both sides. You're going to have to be crafty. You need a set of habits that you can fall back on to create both a new normal, and to dial in to bring yourself back to where you should be.

No matter how busy you are, no matter how many things you have tried and failed, you can do this. It will take a lot of work and sacrifices, but you can get to a healthy weight and stay that way. You don't even have to give up all sweets or your favorite foods forever. But you will have to find a balance that works for you, and know that everything has tradeoffs. Nothing in life is free.

I think by now you've realized that this isn't going to be your typical diet book. A lot of nonfiction books are full of awesome information, with really interesting technical details. However, what often happens is that you read one of those books, get to the very last page, say to yourself "gee, that sure was cool, I know a lot about XYZ now!" And then you live your life exactly that same way you did before the book, because the science or recommendations are a bit too far off for you to actually implement.

This book is focused on implementation. I won't drown you in academic research or horrendously complicated and bland recipes. There is plenty out there that does a great job of that already. My goal isn't to show you the micro details. It is get you executing the macro details and achieving results.

I want to equip you with more things you can do today, rather than fancy scientific terms you have to spend hours on the internet researching. This approach may be less precise, but that is because everyone is different. It may not be the ideal advice for everyone, but I'd argue that decent advice that can be adhered to for years is far superior than great advice that you can only stand to follow for a few weeks.

Most of the time, just knowing the big concepts is plenty. Stop getting bogged down in the detail and get the big things right. If you are looking for more depth on anything in here, jump on Google and go down the rabbit hole. My value add isn't regurgitating miles of information, it is organizing what is important into something that you can read and change your life with.

My end goal is to give you the tools to have the body you want, and to understand how your choices affect your results. I'm not in the business of saying no: I want you to be able to eat what you want, just knowing what you'll have to give up to do so. I don't want you to be the fun-sucker who hasn't eaten a cookie in years, or the worrywart who complains that this cookie will cost 20 minutes on the treadmill. I want you to be the man with the plan, who enjoys the cookie, knowing he has adjusted his next meal for it.

To get there, I'll start off by sharing my background and that of my father, highlighting a few of our biggest lessons learned along the way. Then the focus will shift to actionable things you can start doing right now to make progress, starting with the easiest changes and becoming more intricate as we progress. Finally, I'll zoom back out and talk about how you can keep using this system through a lifetime.

Below is the high level summary things we'll cover over the course of the book:

Consider a diet's sustainability before starting it. Understand what your weight is and what you want it to be. Start by removing refined sugary drinks from your diet. Sleep more and treat sleep as an important factor. Walk more to create a recurring calorie-burning activity. Don't snack between meals. See what intermittent fasting can teach you about hunger. Plan for gradual, lumpy progress. Eat mostly lean meats, veggies, and complex carbohydrates. Eat healthy foods before unhealthy ones (if at all). Cook your own food as much as you can. Don't keep junk food around the house to tempt you. Exercise to build muscle and increase your metabolism.

Keep reading to understand why these are important and how to implement them in your life.

As a disclaimer, nothing in this book is or should be interpreted as medical advice. Everyone should consult with their doctor before beginning any diet or exercise program. Individual medical conditions and needs are something that only a doctor can provide.

CHAPTER 2: INTRO TO HENRY

◆ ◆ ◆

My diet story doesn't take the usual route of a fat kid getting skinny. I have seen both sides of the spectrum, but did it in the reverse order: as a skinny kid getting fat. Having been on both sides of the fence, I want to share the knowledge I gained along the way.

Two things in my life have been constant: regular athletic activity and a fascination with how different diets can improve that athletic activity. I played baseball my entire childhood, and at the end of high school switched to weightlifting as my exercise. I found this to be easier given weightlifting is a solitary activity and not weather-dependent. More interesting, however, has been the dieting that came with it.

When I was ten years old, I stumbled upon one of my dad's Men's Health magazines, found some articles about healthy eating, and immediately became an annoying little kid who refused to eat butter or mayonnaise because they were bad for me. Despite this, at the same time, I had no problem eating pizza and clearly a limited understanding of nutrition. Despite this obvious logical flaw, I became a pretty lean middle schooler. There was one trip, my freshman year of high school, that was a beach trip. I remember doing ab workouts every day for months to get ready for it. I stumbled across the photos recently, and at a waifish 135 pounds, I definitely had abs but was pretty much a stick figure otherwise.

As I got older and into weightlifting to get stronger for baseball, I grew to become a high schooler drinking protein shakes around my workouts. I found bodybuilding magazines and started to learn what I thought was how to get big and strong. This filled in some gaps but still left a lot of holes. By this time, I was about 160 pounds and hoping to turn myself into a power hitter on the baseball field by bulking up. A lot of my friends at the time were either football or hockey players, and so I decided if they could be 200 pounds, I could too.

In the fall of my senior year of high school, I formally declared that I was going to grow from 160 to 200 pounds. I made myself a diet entirely of eating "clean" foods: oatmeal, eggs, lean meats, olive oil, nuts, rice, pasta, bread, and huge amounts of fruit and lean greek yogurt. Game on.

It was the perfect "clean bulk". Eating only healthy foods and doing heavy weightlifting five days per week, I was so excited to magically turn from scrawny to brawny. I was avoiding sugar and unhealthy foods, so knew that I would mostly pack on muscle. The diet began with immediate success. I jumped from probably around 2,000 calories in a full day on my old diet to around 4,000 on the new one.

What was weird was that as I gained weight, my stomach didn't feel softer, but it did protrude more.

"Huh, I guess my abs are growing too," I remember thinking.

One night, after school, I sat down for dinner with my family. I was so full already from the 3,200 or so calories I'd already had that day, but I was not a quitter, so I sat down and buckled up, taking bite after determined bite.

It was grueling. I'd already been chewing all day and was exhausted. Soon, everyone else was done eating. I still had a mountain of food on my plate. My dad and sister left the table, but my mother stayed for moral support. She told me I didn't have to finish it, and that we could just put it in the fridge.

"Never!" was the last thing I croaked before crashing into the table.

I woke up a few hours later with my head on the table to

find my parents laughing at me. Luckily, I had somehow missed the plate when I went down and passed out for two hours. That night, I skipped my after-dinner meal.

Things like this happened a few times. Another time, I spent the entirety of a 90 minute car ride to the Tampa airport trying to eat my way through a gigantic plate of eggs and a bowl of oatmeal. I ashamedly had to throw away the remaining half of my food when we got to the airport.

Despite these struggles, the diet was wildly successful in terms of weight gain. At my peak, I weighed in at 198 in the morning and 207 that night. It definitely wasn't all muscle. I went up a few pant sizes over this time, and as my mom and sister like to point out, gained about ten pounds in my butt and thighs. In my delight at gaining weight, I somehow managed to overlook this.

My parents, in what I think was an attempt to make me see what was actually happening, got me a scale that measured bodyfat that Christmas. Post bulk, I was sitting at around 20% bodyfat. As someone who thought I was all muscle, that was a wakeup call.

I learned a few things I'll never forget on that bulk.

First, eating "clean" doesn't prevent fat gain. It usually makes gaining weight harder, because clean food is usually less calorically dense, but clean food doesn't help if you are still eating too many calories. Just because something is touted as "healthy" does not mean you can't abuse it and make yourself overweight.

Second, when you're getting fat, you often don't recognize it. For example, even though I pride myself on my self-awareness, I was convinced that I was just getting bigger in a good way. What I didn't know is that just like a good steak, as we fatten up, it isn't all in one place. We marble, with a lot of fat mixing in between layers of muscle. Fat won't always be on surface in one spot like you'd expect.

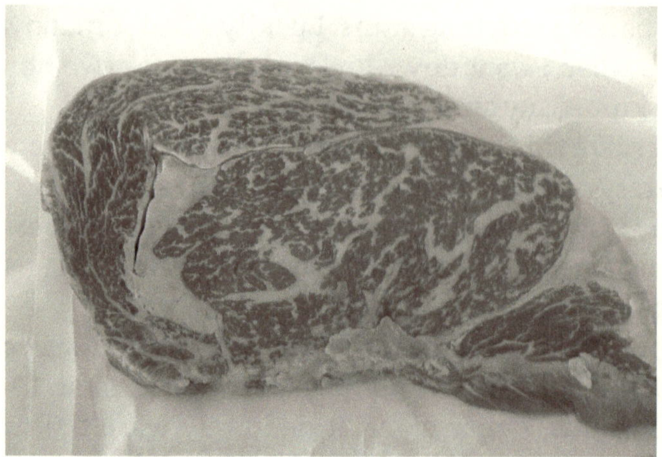

Source: "pic 6236" by BrownGuacamole is licensed under CC BY-ND 2.0

I didn't fully comprehend that my "bulk" had turned into me mostly just getting fatter until one day I ended up seeing myself turned sideways and noticed my gut poking out. I'd always stood facing the mirror, sucking in to hide my belly. The moment I saw how big my belly was sideways without sucking in was jaw-dropping. It had been so easy to deceive myself for so long, giving me an understanding of how many people don't see themselves as they truly are.

The third thing I learned from my bulk was that gaining weight has a snowball effect. Near the end of the bulk, gaining weight got easier. At the beginning, it was exhausting work getting all the food down. But as I got closer to 200 pounds, my hunger grew. I started to crave sweeter foods. Eating wasn't as hard. Once I got through the initial adjustment, my body was happier at the heavier weight and wanted to stay that way.

This was terrifying and convinced me to start cutting weight immediately. At the end of my weight cut, I found myself down to 170 and much happier. Since then, I've oscillated between 160 and 180 depending on my goals and activity. After changing my weight so many times, I've started to notice a lot of patterns. These are what I want to share: the ways I've been able to make changing my weight easier and within my control. I had to learn these lessons the hard way. I hope to share them so you can save yourself the time and do things right the first time.

Mark here - Henry's stories about bulk eating and cutting are true. I didn't approve at the time, and I don't recommend bulk eating for anyone. I was so concerned that I forced Henry to have a physical and full blood work done. He had been eating a dozen or more eggs every-day and I was concerned about his cholesterol. His blood work was fine, only an 18 year old can get away with that. Don't try it!

Now, while I hope these lessons are helpful, I'd be an idiot if I thought that I was the first person to have useful dieting anec-dotes.

Where I bring a different perspective, however, is by com-bining what I've learned about dieting with what I've learned about human behavior from my academic and professional upbringing. I grew up in the world of economics and finance, completing my undergraduate economics degree at Washing-ton University in St. Louis. Post graduation, I completed a pro-fessional designation program in 2018 (the Chartered Financial Analyst curriculum). I currently work on a team within a large asset management firm that focuses on helping people save and invest for a successful retirement.

My undergrad economics courses beat two ideas into me:

First: humans are constantly working to optimize their util-ity (economics-speak for happiness). That means doing things that make us happier, avoiding pain and pursuing pleasure.

Second: everything you do comes at the expense of some-thing else. This is the concept of "opportunity cost" and adds another dimension to optimizing your utility: that the deci-sions you make to optimize your utility mean you are giving up other things.

You can probably guess where this is going: people are bad at making the decisions that truly lead to long-term happiness, and the further they go down the wrong road, the harder it can be to get back on track. The issue is that most people make decisions for short-term utility at the expense of long-term happiness. They also don't account for the opportunity cost: they don't connect the dots between every choice they make.

Beyond just dieting decisions, attitudes and other lifestyle choices have a very real impact on their health. That's pretty bleak, but we have a way to deal with it.

This is where behavioral finance comes in. Behavioral finance is a wonderful, relatively new branch of economics and psychology, that bridges all these vague concepts of "utility" and "opportunity cost" with what people really care about: results.

The gist of behavioral finance is that while traditional economics and finance teach us how the world is in an academic setting, and how people should behave, behavioral finance teaches us how people actually behave: incredibly irrationally.

Traditional finance, or in our case, traditional dieting, assumes that you won't cheat on your diet and eat a box of donuts at 2am because that would hurt your progress and provide disutility. Behavioral finance, or in our case, behavioral dieting, knows that your body is not a rational thing and sometimes just needs to eat those donuts, even if it shouldn't.

We are going to stop pretending we are perfect and learn to outsmart and adapt to our biases, rather than pretending that they don't exist. This is where many traditional diets fail: they assume we are stronger than we are, instead of just accepting us for the weak, irrational creatures we are.

This approach has been paying huge dividends in the real world by helping people save enough to retire, which I see in my current job. You may not read this in the news because it is often underreported, but there is a terrible savings crisis going on in the United States. Many Americans have hardly any savings, and would have to take out a loan to cover even a $400 expense[2]. Some people, in their 50's or 60's and hoping to retire soon, have only a few thousand dollars in their savings accounts[3]. That is not enough to last the rest of their lifetime.

The traditional recommendations to fix this have been things like "save more!", "invest in higher returning assets!" and "find lower fee investments", but the industry has recently come around to the fact that while those behaviors on their own help, they are not nearly enough.

To be truly successful, people need the right things to just happen to them. Doing the right thing has to be as easy as possible, or, when it can be, automatic. To save enough, many people need to be automatically enrolled into a 401(k) account when they start work. Many need automatic escalation in their contributions so that when they earn more money, they automatically save more. They need their company to match part of their savings to encourage them to save more if they want to maximize the match received by their company.

This is because people are amazingly routine-focused and do not make extra time to do things outside of their normal day-to-day activities. That is not to say people are not very smart and driven. The issue is just that we all have our routines that take up all of our time, so it is tough to find an hour to sit down and focus on something that doesn't seem to be that important right now, and to keep revisiting that on a regular basis.

Behavioral finance says "ok fine, we get it, you're busy, we're going to build a system where if you do nothing, you will have the right outcome."

If you transfer this back to dieting, everyone knows that you need to eat veggies and avoid desserts, yet most people don't do nearly enough of this. You need to build a system to make it automatic and easier for yourself to do that. You need a system so that when you fall off the wagon, you can get back on it quickly and painlessly. A system where if you just coast, you will automatically get, or stay, fit and healthy.

That is what we hope to make this book into. We are looking to apply lessons learned in finance, business, and economics to something that everyone can relate to: dieting.

CHAPTER 3: INTRO TO MARK

◆ ◆ ◆

By now you've read the introduction to the book and concepts and Henry's opening chapter on himself. So now a little bit about me, Mark.

As I write this, I'm 57 years old, 31 years older than Henry. I come to our topics from a different direction with a different perspective. As you will see throughout the book, we often agree on recommendations, but not always. Hopefully that will be part of the fun for you as the reader.

I enjoyed a successful career in corporate America, holding Division President roles at three Fortune 500 companies, and later served as President of a large consumer services company. My background has little to do with diet and exercise, but I will make a few connections.

The roles that I worked throughout my career were quite demanding, requiring long hours, extensive travel, and many dreaded client and employee dinners. None of this was good for my waistline! However, my work also enabled me to develop effective skills for problem solving and maintaining discipline - once a goal was chosen.

Let me explain why this book is important to me, which requires a little bit of your patience as I walk through a brief history of my own weight and fitness. I suspect it will be somewhat familiar to many readers.

Throughout high school and college I was reasonably fit and active. My weight was about right for my height and build. I was never much of a formal athlete, but have always been a long fast walker and backpacked extensively while in college.

After college, I hit the ground running in the workforce, regularly working 12 hour days when you include commuting time. That left me with little time and even less motivation for diet and exercise. Thanks to the faster metabolism that a typical male enjoys in his 20's, I only gained a few pounds or so in those years.

In my early 30's, both of my children were born. This was a treacherous time for maintaining weight. My work stilled chewed up 12 hours of each day, and I wanted to spend the little free time I had with the kids, not exercising. The bigger challenge was all of the food in the house all the time. My wife did an amazing job preparing healthy and tasty food for the children, but the unintended consequence was that I was eating more than my share.

By my late 30's, I was about 10 pounds over the top recommendation of the height and weight chart for my height (much more on this later). The obvious and technical label for this condition was "overweight". Despite my weight, most people would have described me as "skinny" at the time. This was the first of 2 weight peaks in my life.

At the end of my 30's, my career took a very positive turn, and I was sent to Singapore for what was intended to be a two year stint. Shortly after relocating myself and the family, I was promoted to president for all of Asia for my employer and stayed for eight years. I was running a portfolio of over 40 different companies spread across 12 countries with combined revenues exceeding $1 billion. As the reader will imagine, I traveled 3 ½ weeks per month and maintained a grueling schedule. So much for controlled diet and exercise.

Throughout Asia, it is a business norm for host companies to entertain visiting executives every night. With very few exceptions over the eight years I was in Asia, I never ate dinner alone and was rarely back to my hotel room before 11:00 PM. I also ate a hotel breakfast and lunch out everyday as well.

The funny thing though: overall, while in Asia and through my 40's, my weight dropped by about 12-15 pounds from my USA high.

I thought I was thin, but nope, just less fat.

The simple reason for my weight loss was that the portions in Asia were smaller. A true "a ha" moment for me occurred in 2004, when for a combination of business reasons, I had not been back in the US for close to 2 years. I then traveled back to Denver, Colorado for a business conference. My country manager for Malaysia was traveling with me. We arrived in Denver later in the afternoon after 30 hours of transit time from the other side of the world. Too tired to think very hard about dinner, we walked out of our hotel intending to grab dinner at someplace close and convenient.

As it turns out, the restaurant we selected was a famous chain fast casual restaurant. We each ordered something typical like nachos and chicken fingers. When our food arrived, in my mind's eye, it was served piled high on plates the size of garbage can lids. We both laughed until we cried. The US portions were shockingly large and it took a multi year absence from the US for me to notice. My colleague and I were in agreement that in Asia, our two entrees would have easily served 10 people.

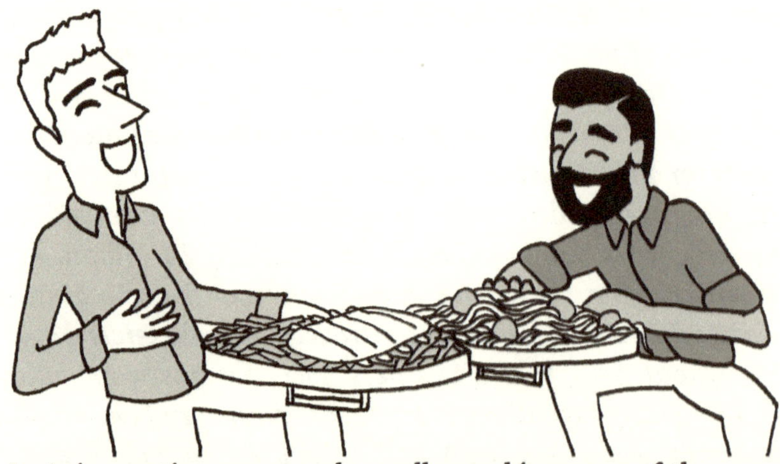

In Asia, portions are much smaller and in many of the countries with ethnic Chinese heritage, food is typically served family style, often on rotating platters on round tables. Each guest at dinner takes his or her portion of each dish, with chopsticks, from a shared platter. That makes it hard to load 5,000 calories onto your plate in a socially acceptable way.

Before I left Asia, despite the challenging work and lack of work-life balance, I did manage to stay in decent shape by doing 14 kilometer run/hikes through the Singapore jungle most Sunday afternoons and mountain biking with Henry in a "secret jungle area" of Singapore that was accessed from a trail hidden off the side of a highway exit ramp. It also happened to be an infrequently used training area for the Singapore military. On the few occasions that we met soldiers in training, they were very polite about our trespassing.

At the age of 46, I returned with my family to the US. My new US-based job included international responsibility for a number of companies and I continued to travel extensively around the world. Slowly, between 2008 and 2014, my weight crept back up to the same peak I had reached in my 30's. The Asia impact of smaller portions had finally worn off.

So, at the age of 52, 13 pounds over the top of the "normal" range for my height, I starting to experience the symptoms of GERDS (gastroesophageal reflux disease), mostly heartburn.

I've been very fortunate health-wise throughout my life. I don't take any prescriptions and my medical results have always been in healthy ranges. But, with the GERDS-like symptoms, I immediately researched the internet and then went to the drug store and purchased a package each of all three of the leading over-the-counter heartburn medications and started popping pills. They more or less worked and relieved the symptoms. However, I was pretty unhappy with myself and didn't want to start taking maintenance medication for the rest of my life. After much reading, I decided to lose a few pounds to see if that would help.

It did. After losing 5 pounds, the GERDS symptoms disappeared entirely! No more medications for me. I proceeded to lose a total of 28 pounds over the next two months and have held to that weight for 5 years and counting. How I was able to lose the excess weight and maintain an ideal weight is the story that I want to share. It wasn't too hard. Often, it was fun, and the positive comments I received were a great reward for the effort.

My commitment to maintaining an optimal weight has become a passion and a self competition for me. A competition where winning is not just great for its own sake, but will likely lead to a longer and healthier life.

CHAPTER 4: MAGIC
ISN'T REAL

◆ ◆ ◆

"Look at you, with your fancy abs!"

Either my mother or sister said it. An offhand comment to them, but it meant the world to me. It was the first time I can recall someone in my family telling me I was in great shape. The fact that they noticed me being fitter than normal meant that I had made true progress, not just "I look better with the right lighting progress".

This little comment led to the wonderful feeling you can only get from achieving something that can't be bought and you have to earn yourself. I was 20 years old, back from my junior year of college on winter break. I had been slowly cutting weight since August, little by little, until I got to "fancy abs" level. I was weighing around 170, and I had veins in my lower stomach, and one running up my side oblique, yet I still held a significant amount of muscle mass. I looked like I lifted weights and was ready for a beach photoshoot. Even without flexing, in any lighting, my abs were clear as day, and I was ecstatic about it.

My ego was stroked even more when I walked through town to the beach with my shirt off. I was going to walk along the shoreline to decompress from a tough semester at school. As I strolled through the Village on Siesta Key, people turned their heads to take a second look at me. A few women and college girls yelled playful catcalls as I went by. At one point, a woman even yelled out of a car "dayum!" as she drove by. I could see my muscle definition through car and storefront windows as I walked through town.

I felt like a movie star. It was exactly what I'd always imagined being ripped would feel like. I was on top of the world. The six years of lifting and obsessing about my diet had paid off.

By the time I got to the beach, I was half expecting a Hollywood or fitness model talent scout to approach me and ask if I'd be interested in doing some work. I was waiting for some bombshell actress to approach me, introduce herself, and suddenly become my girlfriend.

None of that happened.

I just kept walking, for hours, stressing about normal college student things: how I did on midterms and wondering what my friends were up to. Before long, I'd almost entirely forgotten about the walk through town. I may have had "fancy abs" like I'd always wanted, but nothing different happened. The heavens didn't part. All of my wildest dreams didn't come true. Sure, people noticed, and occasionally made comments, but otherwise, it was just a normal day.

Despite getting to the body composition I'd always dreamed of, it quickly started to feel empty. My abs hadn't cured every other problem in my life, and I felt foolish when I realized that I had subconsciously believed that they would. Achieving this look, with the leanness and muscularity, had always been an epic goal I had been chasing, but once I got there, I found it to be a mirage. If I wanted success in other areas of life, I would still have to work at those. Things were not just going to happen to me now that I was in great shape.

More interestingly, despite being in a place where most people would be happy to stay in for the rest of their lives, I wanted more. I'd reached my goal, and suddenly that wasn't enough. The goalposts moved, and I wanted to be this lean but with more muscle mass. Before long, I was purposefully gaining weight again to get stronger, and just like that, the fancy abs were gone.

Months later, after gaining a bit of muscle mass, I cut weight again, trying to re-live the "fancy abs". It didn't quite work out. I didn't have something dialed in right, and wasn't as muscular the next time. Very lean, but looking almost scrawny rather than as good as I did in December. The fact that I had done it before didn't mean I was guaranteed to do it again.

I share this story because it taught me, in multiple ways, that "magic isn't real". This sounds like a nuance that matters little compared to the nitty gritty details of actually getting fit. In the short term, it is just a small nuance, but over the course of a lifetime, understanding this concept will lead you to a much more pleasant and productive path to fitness. Magic not being real is most clearly explained in three different ways: magic life-changes, magic maintenance, and magic foods.

Magic Life Changes

As I quickly learned after my beach walk, getting fit will not, on its own, result in your entire life changing into a fairytale. Yes, you will be more healthy, and by many standards, more attractive. Yes, putting in the work and discipline to transform your body will make you more organized and focused, which will help you in other aspects of life. But to be clear, if you are a jerk, you will just turn into a fit jerk. If you are lazy at your job, you will just be a fit lazy employee. If you are too shy to make friends, you will just be fit and shy. You will still have bills to pay, abs or no abs. Your other faults will not be magically erased by your fitness, so don't plan on getting in shape to be the key to changing your life.

That is not to say it won't be helpful. For many people, myself included, fitness is a hobby that makes them healthier and happier and helps them succeed in other areas of life. Just know that it is only one facet of a full and successful life. Do not assume that focusing on your fitness alone is enough. If you have other problems, your abs won't solve them. You have to solve them.

In fact, for many people, their obsession with fitness and inability to be flexible with their rules and diets creates new problems. I'd be lying if I said I had never been one of these people. My urging to you, reader, is to make fitness a part of your life, rather than making it everything in your life. This book aims to show you how you can do that.

Mark here - Henry doesn't quite say it, but changing your appearance and physique is something you do for yourself, not to solicit compliments from others. Make the changes solely for you and relish the stray compliments that may come. That said, the self-confidence gained from being in control of your body and choices can influence your life in other positive ways.

Magic Maintenance

Many people follow excruciatingly difficult diets for a short time period because they are certain that once they get the results they want, everything will be easy. This isn't the case. If you try to create shortcuts to long term results, you are likely just kicking the can down the road.

Once you hit your goal, rainbows will not appear in the distance, and angels will not start singing. The world will not irrevocably change for you now that you have the body you've been working towards. Your new body won't miraculously become impossibly easy to maintain. The rules of the universe won't change now that you finally have the physique you want. This was a slap in the face for me when I discovered that just because I had that awesome physique once didn't guarantee I could keep it, or easily get back to it.

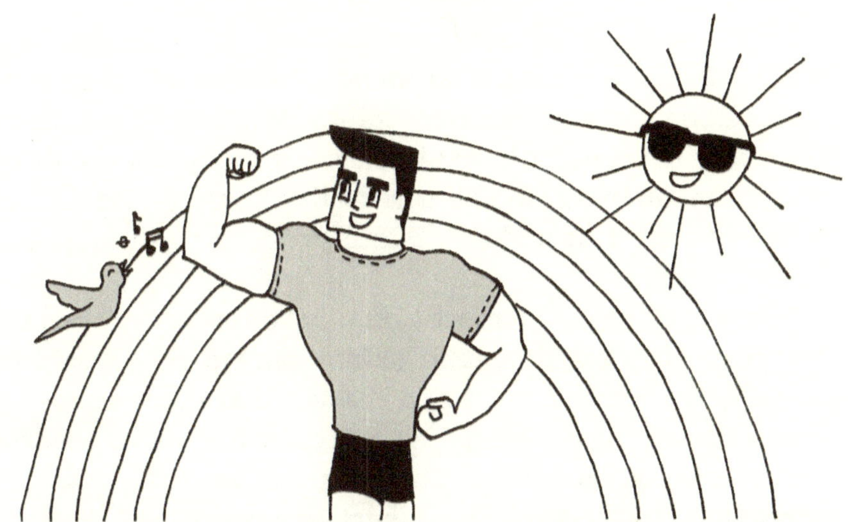

Temptations and roadblocks will always exist. Even if you know exactly how to maintain your physique, life obstacles will still rear their ugly heads and derail you. You'll go on a vacation where the only food you can eat is pasta or scones, and you'll gain weight. You'll get invited to a bachelor(ette) party where you eat and drink your way through a city. You'll be at a business convention where the only food is little sandwiches for three days. Sometimes you can't avoid those things, and you may get off track. Your physique will not maintain itself perfectly as it was at your peak. That is normal.

This happens to people all the time. See almost every Hollywood actor who buffed up to play a superhero and then returned to a normal physique a few months later. Yes, part of that may be due to chemical assistance, but the point remains: few people achieve perfect bodies and maintain them indefinitely.

That is called life. Plan for it.

All doom and gloom aside, maintaining your physique will be easier than it was to get in the first place. It will take work, but once you can dial your body in around a set weight, it will be relatively comfortable hovering around that weight.

Magic Foods

You've seen the advertisements. The one fruit that is the healthiest thing on the planet for you. That supplement everyone is taking. I won't even list specifics, because by the time I do, something new will be around. The names vary, but the story is always the same: this food burns fat like nothing else on earth. Eat a little bit of it and all of your problems will melt away. That's a fantasy.

Salads are one of the most egregious offenders of the magic food ploy. They are the classic "skinny-person" food, yet you've probably started to catch on to the fact that many salads have more calories than normal foods. Even worse, many that have less calories do so because they don't have enough satiating macronutrients, leaving you hungry so you end up bingeing on ice cream late at night. This isn't to say that all salads are bad, just that you should take a closer look at them before unquestioningly accepting that they are healthier than regular meals.

Regardless of what the exact magic food or supplement is, people's thought process is often similar: now that they are eating it, they are covered, so the rest of their diet is fine and above scrutiny.

Wrong. Everything matters. Eating a few "superfoods" will not cancel out the bad ones you eat after them. Eating spinach and a cheeseburger may mean you're getting a serving of veggies, but you're still having a cheeseburger.

You will have dramatically better results eating mediocre foods in the proper quantities than throwing a few "magic foods" into a poorly portioned diet.

That's not to say that some foods will not help you on your journey - there certainly are clear choices that will make an impact. However, you can't just eat them on top of a bad diet and call it a day. They have to be one piece of a larger plan.

Everything Matters

This leads us back to one of the main principles of the book: you have to attack your health and fitness from as many angles as you can, because you may lose the ability or interest in one angle at any given time. We are looking to maximize your probability and longevity of results, so we have to put our eggs in multiple baskets.

Dieting and changing your physique can be done quickly and effectively, but it isn't just a walk in the park where at the end you never have to pay attention to what you eat again. If you are going to be successful and remain successful, you need a mindset shift, not a quick solution.

Most people go astray by living as if they are just on the brink of one of these fitness fairytales, where they make a few good choices and immediately become a cover model. This leads to them looking for quick fixes, which makes trying to get in shape an even more uphill battle than it already is.

You can't just assume that the battle ends when you hit your goal. Staying fit is a lifelong endeavor, where you will fight the same battles over and over again for years. You need to build in a plan that you won't hate for the long haul, or you've lost before you've even begun.

This means making sure your diet and fitness routine is something that is satisfying to you, and doesn't disrupt everything else in your life. It has to be sustainable, which is what we will explore in the next chapter.

CHAPTER 5: MAKE IT SMALL AND SUSTAINABLE

◆ ◆ ◆

It was our sophomore year night out. I was 19 years old, and we had all just returned to Washington University in St. Louis ("WashU") after summer break. The student government had allocated funds to rent out Blueberry Hill, a St. Louis landmark. Decked out with memorabilia photos of celebrities who have visited over the years, Blueberry Hill sat in the middle of the Loop, a street just north of WashU packed with bars and restaurants frequented by locals, college students, and tourists.

Chuck Berry, singer of "Johnny b Goode," which was immortalized as the essence of rock and roll in the classic movie Back to the Future, was a St. Louis resident who often performed at Blueberry Hill. Though I knew he was well into in his 90's, I had hoped Chuck would make an appearance that night.

It was around eight o'clock, and my friends were getting ready to go head over. As I got my shoes on and got ready to join them, it hit me: I hadn't eaten since five. The all-important three hour mark was about to hit, and I was sure that I was at risk of going into catabolism. That meant my muscles, which hadn't had protein in hours, would start to waste away, and all the gains I'd been working so hard towards in the gym would melt into oblivion.

Not on my watch. I had planned for this.

I grabbed a tub of cottage cheese, a plastic fork, and a paper towel, and caught up to the group. We walked across campus to the Loop, sharing stories of our summer adventures and speculating on who would be there tonight. I munched through my 16 ounce tub of cottage cheese as we went, loving every bite.

"You can't bring that in." The bouncer scowled at me when we arrived.

"What do you mean? It's just cottage cheese! This is a school event. What's the problem?"

After a few volleys, we got nowhere. It became clear that I had two options: toss the cottage cheese in the trash, or finish eating it outside and then come in.

Enraged that they were raining on my parade but determined to get my protein in, I sat on the curb until I had finished the whole tub. One of my friends was nice enough to wait for ten minutes with me while I finished eating before we went in and went on with our night.

This kind of ridiculousness didn't end with the cottage cheese. One of my other specialties was my infamous "pocket chicken". We'd be in the middle of class, the library, or a hiking trip - really anywhere - and I would pull out of my pocket a piece of baked chicken breast, slimy from condensation and as white as sand. It was pure protein. I couldn't help myself: it was just so convenient. People around me were quite grossed out, and I don't think anyone ever asked me for a bite. My buddies still give me crap about the pocket chicken.

Looking back, I try not to consider the social damage it must have done to be that kid carrying around his cottage cheese and pocket chicken. Yet what fascinates me is that while that was ridiculous four years ago, it has become more mainstream now. Plenty of people are paleo, or gluten free, or organic-only now, and it has become more socially acceptable to be on a diet so excruciatingly annoying that you can't go anywhere anymore.

This is ridiculous. Like me a few years ago, those that are so obsessive about their diet that they have to carry outside food everywhere are likely overdoing it. Most people other than competitive athletes or those preparing for a physique competition do not need to go to this extreme. If you are just trying to get in better shape, this level of OCD with your food is overkill.

Being this intense with your diet may work, but likely will become so difficult to maintain over time that you will fall off the wagon. Most diets work in the short term, but then again, all sorts of crazy things work in the short term. You can drive 100 miles per hour to work - you'll get there really fast for a day, or maybe even a week, until the cops pull you over and slow down your party. A lot of diets are like that: they work, but only for a short time, and then you're back to square one.

There is only so long you can be on a diet that is incredibly difficult before you decide "screw it" and go back to your old ways. To address this, I believe we need a new definition of a successful diet. The term "diet" itself misses half the picture. We need a system of eating, living and exercising that we can practice for the rest of our lives. A system that is easy enough that we don't have to obsess over the details, giving us time to do what is important to us. This goes back to the behavioral finance element: we need to set things up like a 401(k), so that the automatic option, the path of least resistance, pushes us in the right direction.

To use a different investing metaphor, everyone wants to find the diet that is like a high return hedge fund. They want the fund with huge returns every year that will make them rich without them having to save more money. These funds exist, but they are rare, and most are either not available for new investors or only maintain good performance for a few years. Many end up exploding spectacularly. Investing in one is a burden that requires continuous monitoring and expertise to make sure the fund is doing what it is supposed to. High-intensity, complicated diets are the same way - sometimes they work very well, but often they backfire and lead people to extreme binges or swearing off dieting all together.

For most people, the magic hedge fund solution will not

work. A far more effective solution to build wealth, with a higher probability of success, is the un-exciting practice of consistently saving for many years. Dieting is the same way: a set of fundamental habits they can repeatedly fall back on over the long term will be far more effective than a hyper-effective diet they can only sustain for a few months.

To do this, we're going to focus on implementation. I'd like to introduce the Diet Sustainability Matrix. This is something I've come up with as a way to judge whether a diet can be sustained for more than just a few weeks. Save yourself a lot of pain and before you jump on the paleo organic keto vegan diet train, or whatever trend hits the magazines next month, see if the diet you are about to try is sustainable across these five dimensions:

First, socially sustainable: Is it a pain to do in social situations? Does it annoy people around you? Does it inconvenience people preparing food for you?

Second, financially sustainable: Does it require costly ingredients outside your budget? Do you have to buy new diet resources on a regular basis to find out what you should be eating?

Third, psychologically sustainable: Does it permanently ban foods that are important to you? Does it require you to regularly eat things you find vile? Does it make you constantly miserable for long periods of time (outside of initial break-in periods?) Does it make you constantly worry about what you're eating to a degree that is detrimental to your life?

Fourth, logistically sustainable: Does it require an unreasonable amount of time to prepare or eat food? Is it possible to do while traveling or eating out? Does it require rare or hard to find ingredients?

Finally, lifetime sustainable: Is it flexible enough to do across different life phases? Is it flexible enough to be usable whether you are moderately losing weight to be healthier, aggressively losing weight to be very lean, maintaining weight, or attempting to gain weight?

Not all diets will check all boxes, or even a majority of boxes on the sustainability matrix. That doesn't mean they suck, it just means you will probably only be able to do them for a short period of time.

You may be frustrated because you just realized that the diet you want to do does not meet the five criteria. Perhaps you want to do a 6 week extreme diet to get that last few ounces of body fat off, or need to gain weight and eat six meals per day to do so. Do that, reap the benefits, and come back to your system that fits the sustainability matrix.

Think of the sustainability matrix as a guideline for what the diet you design as your home base. Your home base diet should meet all or almost all criteria on the sustainability matrix, and is one you can come back to and do for years at a time without psychological hardship. If you need to have a few weeks of insanity of some diet that doesn't meet all the sustainability matrix, go for it, but know that you'll revert to your home base diet over the long run.

A decade is five hundred and twenty weeks. That is over 86 six week stretches. That is 3,640 days. Even if you have the perfect diet, if it only lasts six weeks, in the long run, it is useless. What matters more is the diet you come back to after you quit the six week diet: the diet you can stay on for decades.

Put Down the Bazooka, Champ

Many diets don't work for people because they pack way too much firepower. Odds are that you don't need to resort to eating kale and egg whites every meal, you just need to make a few lifestyle changes. Why would you start with the hard stuff when you can tackle the easy stuff first?

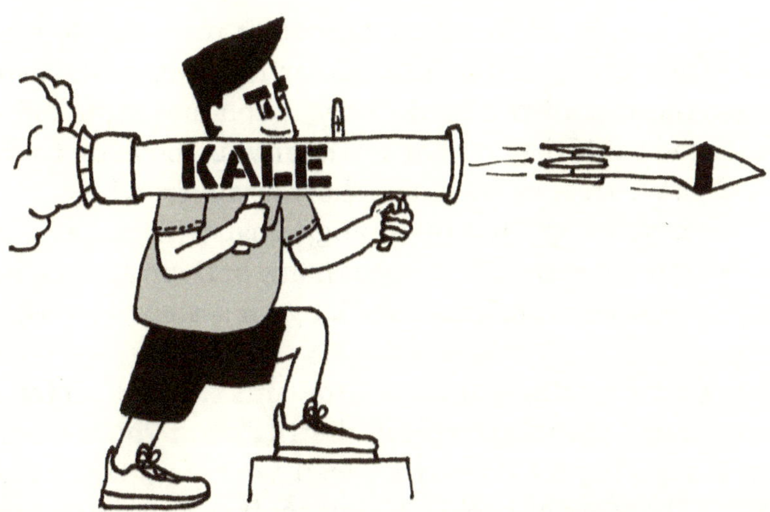

As a species, we don't have as much willpower as we might think. A lot of it is used up making tough decisions at our jobs and in our family lives, so not much remains to help us stay strong against diet demons. You can try to be a hero and grind everything out with willpower, or you can play smarter and work on making tiny changes that you can sustain for the rest of your life, and then you can almost not worry about dieting and go back to living a fun life.

How do you do that? Start small. One change at a time. Change is hard and scary, so don't go overboard at once. Keeping it to one change also gives you two benefits. First, it lets you isolate your variables and figure out if the change made an impact. Second, it leaves you to make more changes whenever you stop benefitting from the first change. That way, you can continue to gradually steer your body in the right direction, instead of just shocking it quickly. As we'll get into later in the book, if you try to make too dramatic changes, your body will reject them and you may not make any progress at all.

You don't need to diet like a fitness model. You just need to diet like a slightly skinnier version of yourself. You need to keep doing that until you continue to make progress and, if it is your goal, until a slightly skinnier version of yourself is a fitness model.

The book is ordered in a very deliberate manner. We start with the easiest changes. If those work for you, keep doing them and forget the rest of the book. Why spend any more effort than you need to? If they do not work for you, move on to the next section. We are looking to find shortcuts everywhere, both within our psychology and physiology, that will make being lean just a little bit easier. We want as many of them as possible, so you can minimize your effort and let your system do most of the work.

Things get increasingly involved towards the end, which is where you'll find the more typical "dieting" stuff you were expecting. If any chapter doesn't sit well with you, that's fine: don't do it. These are just tools in your toolkit. You are the one that has to try them out and see what works for you. Our goal is just to show you the spectrum of instruments you have to work with, and things that are likely making a big impact on your body composition efforts.

You may find that you come back to this book for another read and see things in a totally different light. Some things that felt ridiculous the first time you read it may resonate the second time. Your body changes along with your mind. Don't be too surprised if some of these techniques work better than others for you, and if what works changes over time.

Mark here - Henry is the most self-disciplined person I've met, he can develop and follow a rule set with relative ease. If all of the above is a bit daunting, a very simple rule you could follow is "eat less and eat less often".

CHAPTER 6: KNOW THY BELLY

◆ ◆ ◆

For some reason, men are incredibly bad at assessing whether they are overweight. Women are usually very self-aware of and self-conscious about their bodies, but men often swing dramatically in the other direction. In the US, it seems almost inevitable that when you enter your thirties and forties, you are destined for the "dad bod". Fit middle-aged men are the exception in most places, and this seems to be socially accepted. What gives?

For much of my life, I've been puzzled by the link between masculinity and unhealthy foods. Beer, hamburgers, fries, and big fatty steaks are "manly", while salads are "girly". To me, this has always been counterintuitive because eating these "manly" foods makes you overweight, slow, unhealthy, and physically unattractive to many people.

Before you complain and say that people like less lean guys, why is it that so many romantic adult novels have shirtless guys with abs on the covers? Why don't they have pudgy guys on the covers? Clearly, the masses have spoken and they want the covers with the ripped guys.

So men are not eating these foods to attract romantic attention. It just seems to be something that is culturally accepted. I have two broad theories as to why. We'll call them the "calories are manly" and "weight is power" theories.

Calories are Manly Theory

A few centuries ago, most men spent their days outside, farming, fighting, or building things with their hands. It was tough, energy-intensive work that sometimes involved not eating for long stretches of time. If men didn't get enough calories in at every chance, they might either see dramatic drops in job performance or actually have ill health effects from being undernourished. "Manly" activities require a lot of calories. To quantify this, take a look at the calories burned per hour at a few different jobs[4]:

Job	Calories Per Hour
Light Office Work	34
Carpentry, General	170
Farming, Shoveling Grain	306
Coal Mining, General	340
Forestry, General	476

Assuming an eight hour day, you would only need 272 calories of nourishment to make up for the work you did if you were an office worker. However, if you were a carpenter, you'd need 1,360 calories, and using a more extreme example, if you were a logger performing forestry, you'd need 3,808 calories.

These examples are unrealistically precise, but directionally prove an important point: people in the past, with manual labor jobs, simply had to eat as many calories as possible to stay alive. That meant the full burger, fries, and beer, or whatever the equivalent.

Hundreds of years ago, if you could get away with eating salad at every meal, that meant that you simply weren't doing any hard work, which would surely be looked at as unmanly. If you were caught at a logging cabin eating a spinach salad, you'd be laughed out of the room, and with good reason: you wouldn't have enough calories to actually get the job done and would be a liability to the team.

Fast forward to today, and men still get laughed at by other men for eating "girly" low calorie foods, except most of these men now work in sedentary office jobs. The culture hasn't yet caught up to the environment, and as a result, many men are overweight.

Weight is Protection Theory

All things equal, if you pit two animals against each other in a fight, the bigger one will usually win. This applies to people as well, and is why boxing has weight classes: a 200 pound person is generally stronger than a 160 pound person. Up to a point, people who weigh more, especially those exercising, have more muscle mass, making them stronger. Not only that, but body fat can provide protection from blows and cuts that a very lean person wouldn't get. For example, archaeologists have speculated that ancient gladiators were fed a carb-heavy diet because "a fat cushion protects you from cut wounds and shields nerves and blood vessels in a fight[5]."

Generally, with animals, those in the wild with access to more food become bigger, more dominant, and end up having higher social status because of their physical power. I believe a similar scenario happened for humans in previous centuries, especially in eras where they were doing primarily manual labor or combat jobs. The additional calories would help them get larger and stronger, and their high activity levels would help them build muscle and keep them from becoming debilitatingly fat. They then became the most productive workers, or strongest warriors, giving them advantages in their society.

In past centuries, even those that did become incredibly fat were respected because while they didn't have the physical power and speed, the fact that they had enough wealth to not have to do tough manual labor, and enough food to actually get that fat, showed that they were truly rich.

I believe these historical benefits of being heavier still reside in masculine culture, and lead us to an environment where men think chicken and light beer are for sissies.

Had this been any other century, they would have been right, but things have changed in today's world. We no longer live in the wild: most of us live in captivity. Most people have desk jobs and can't possibly burn off enough calories with the few hours of exercise they can fit in before and after work to eat only calorie-dense food like their ancestors did. Now, almost everyone has access to enough food to weigh as much as they want, so if you weigh a lot it just means you weigh a lot, not that you are a rich king.

Yet one nuance hasn't changed: being physically powerful and muscular still confers an advantage. It is just much harder to get there today since most of our jobs don't incorporate exercise, and we are surrounded by processed, fattening foods. Men still know they want to be big and strong, but can't disassociate that with the "manly" foods that used to be necessary to get there. Today's challenge is being big and manly while still being lean and having limited time to work out. To do that, men need to eat a much more traditional "healthy diet".

I will discuss exercise in slightly more detail in a later chapter, but generally won't address building muscle elsewhere in the book because there are already dozens of great resources on that.

I recognize that my argument for manly foods is relatively abstract, so let's focus on something that happens all the time: men who are athletes in high school and college often define their identity around their athletic build ("I'm six-four and 225 pounds"). After they stop playing, they keep that identity, and decide they want to maintain their playing weight. They stay the same weight for decades, but instead of working out like a varsity athlete, they get a few short gym sessions in a few times per week. Their muscles atrophy, but they keep eating the same, so their weight stays the same. Over time, they develop a belly, but their brains have trouble processing that they are fat because they still fit in their pants and don't weigh any more than they used to.

Or, even more frustrating, is the trap I mentioned in my introduction: men who decide they want to get brawny and successfully gain weight, but are unable to realize that a lot of the weight they have gained is fat.

Many men have fallen into these traps. You can get out, but if you are going to, you need to really understand how far you need to go. You may find that you have been dishonest with yourself, so this may hurt.

A warning before you continue. The exercise that follows is not meant to be demeaning, but a wakeup call to those in the trap of self-illusion. If you already feel self-conscious about your body and understand the progress you need to make, you can skip the next few paragraphs until you get to my dad's section.

The Mirror

Go to a private room with the biggest mirror you can find. Take your shirt off. Look at yourself. Turn sideways and keep looking. Like what you see? If you do, that might be about to change. Close your eyes. Take five slow, deep breaths, and try to relax every muscle in your body. Open your eyes and look at yourself but stay just as relaxed. You'll find that suddenly you aren't subconsciously sucking your stomach in this time. Keep looking, and keep that stomach relaxed. Now, turn sideways again but keep your stomach muscles relaxed. Seeing a different picture than you did before?

We're going to take things one step farther. Go to another private room without a mirror. Get a camera that can do video recording. Turn it on and perch it somewhere that has a full view of you. Look at the camera, and do the relaxation exercise. Do a full three hundred and sixty degree turn, stopping at each ninety degree angle and relaxing your stomach for a few breaths.

Now, go look at the video. You might be surprised by what you see. Your body, without the benefit of you subtly finding the best lighting and poses that you would in the mirror, may not be all you thought it was. You may be a bit wider than you thought. Most people, especially those of us that are not truly fat but just a few pounds overweight, hide it well, especially from the front.

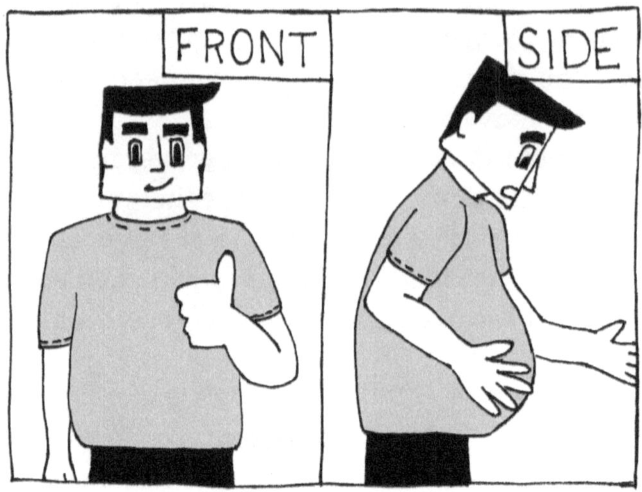

Men are especially good at hiding their stomachs from themselves. Men can often grow a sizable gut before their actual waist size increases, since for men, fat often accumulates right above the belt line in a delightful belly overhang. This is how you can see men that look 8 months pregnant but still wear size 33 pants. If you have this, it can be hard to see from the front, and when you turn sideways, your body can't help but suck in so you don't notice that you're a little wider than you see yourself.

I am victim to this on a regular basis. Usually every year, I decide to "bulk" up to get stronger for lifting. I end up gaining ten to twenty pounds and feeling awesome because I get stronger and think I am the hulk. Suddenly, I fill out shirts better and my arms feel huge. Yet once the bulk is over, I always cut weight to get a little bit leaner and make the muscle mass more visible. Every single time, after losing a few pounds on the cut, I realize that I had actually been fatter than I had realized and just hid it behind bigger muscles. This happens year after year without fail.

After the mirror exercise, you have just seen yourself as you truly are, maybe for the first time. This is important because it breaks down the barrier between how you see yourself, and what other people see, which is what actually exists. If there is no difference between what you thought you'd see and what you actually saw when relaxing, congratulations: you are in a small minority. If you were surprised and unhappy with what you saw, join the club.

It might hurt right now. That is ok. If you aren't happy with where you are, use this as motivation. Keep the video and watch it months from now when you are lighter. You are no longer kidding yourself, and now likely know that you need to make some changes. Reality might have just smacked you in the face. Take some time to soak it in, and when you're done mourning for your shattered reality, let's go to the next step: figuring out how much you should weigh, and measuring yourself.

Quick aside - if you are demoralized right now, skip ahead to the "Why are you doing this?" chapter and come back. It will help motivate you.

Mark here - Henry started this chapter with the provocative title of "Know thy belly." In my words, let's determine the right weight for you. Face it, you weigh too much and you know it.

You wouldn't be reading this book if you thought you were at the ideal weight. I keep reading various statistics stating that a frighteningly high percentage of adults in the US are obese. There seems to be a plethora of evidence that indicates that being obese will shorten your lifespan, and I think as or more importantly, shorten your healthspan, which I will define as the years of your life that you are healthy enough and fit enough to travel, play with children, enjoy your hobbies and just be active. Being fat and sick is not something to aspire to. If you aren't obese, but overweight, you still may be pretty unhappy with yourself in the mirror. The purpose of this section is to guide you to find your ideal weight. Get ready. It may be a shock!

I've already made a glancing reference to standard height and weight charts. Basically, they list a weight range for each inch of height. The height and weight charts directly correlate to the BMI calculation and range.

Before we look at the tables, let's talk about BMI for a minute.

The standard healthy range is frequently quoted as being between 19 and 24, overweight between 25 and 30, and over 30 as being obese. The BMI range quoted is fairly consistent across quite a few height and weight charts. The chart shown below is easy to understand and doesn't differ according to gender or weight. Pounds are pounds.

Said another way, a pound of muscle weighs the same as a pound of fat. I left off the BMI of 19 column because I think 19 is unrealistically skinny. I left a space for separation but did include the 25 column. If your weight is in the 25 column and you look amazing, congratulations, you must be very fit! Also note that data on this chart is from 1998, before the obesity crisis was largely recognized. Some of the more recent tables have values that have been expanded, just like our waistlines!

Let's determine your ideal weight.

Below are you are looking at weight values that correlate to BMI values between 20 and 25. Two additional factors now need to be considered, your relative frame size and your muscularity. Note that the chart doesn't differentiate between men and women, but frame size and muscularity does differ. Here is an informal methodology to choose the correct weight for yourself.

BMI	20	21	22	23	24	25
	<	<	Weight	>	>	
Height						
4'11"	99	104	109	114	119	124
5'	102	107	112	118	123	128
5'1"	106	111	116	122	127	132
5'2"	109	115	120	126	131	136
5'3"	113	118	124	130	135	141
5'4"	116	122	128	134	140	145
5'5"	120	126	132	138	144	150
5'6"	124	130	136	142	148	155
5'7"	127	134	140	146	153	159
5'8"	131	138	144	151	158	164
5'9"	135	142	149	155	162	169
5'10"	139	146	153	160	167	174
5'11"	143	150	157	165	172	179
6"	147	154	162	169	177	184
6'1"	151	159	166	174	182	189
6'2"	155	163	171	179	186	194
6'3"	160	168	176	184	192	200

The exact middle range is at 22 BMI. If you are male, start at the 23 column. If you are female, start at the 21 column. If you have a large frame (think about foot and hand size, because they don't accumulate fat) go up a column. If you have a small frame, go down a column.

Do the same for muscularity - your call on how to define, but don't lie to yourself. If you are truly heavier due to muscles and think you should be at a weight higher than the model I've presented, I have a test for you. At the weight I'm recommending, you are likely to see at least an outline of abs, I don't mean a sculpted 6 pack, but at least a good outline. If you can't see abs at the weight you think is right, try my weight calculation instead.

Here is my real life example. I am a 5'8" male, my frame is on the small side and I consider myself fit, but not heavily muscled. So I start at a value of 23 BMI, subtract 1 for my frame and no adjustment for muscularity. My ideal weight is at 22 BMI, 144 pounds for my height. Based on experience, I know this exactly right for me.

This should be your normal baseline weight. This is the weight you get back to after food bingeing (big nights out, corporate events, super bowl parties, game day in general). I recommend that you get back to your baseline weight after each food binge (before the next binge occurs!). That said, my typical weight ranges between 146 and 147, so 2 -3 pounds over ideal. Just enough to hide those abs!

Henry again here - if you are like some of my weightlifting buddies who read this chapter, you are probably scoffing because you have a high BMI but do have abs. I want to reiterate: this is possible for some people who carry a lot of muscle mass. BMI generally has a high inverse correlation with leanness, but that is not always the case. If you are one of the heavily muscled exceptions to this, feel free to raise your target weight to line up with where it should be.

That said, if you are an exception to this rule, I challenge you: how lean are you actually? A lot of weightlifters are relatively lean, but if they ever try to cut weight to get really lean, they find that instead of losing the 10 pounds of fat they thought they had, they lost 20 or 30. You may not be as lean as you think, so don't knock the BMI table until you do a true weight cut and see how heavy you are at your leanest. Personally, I range between 23 and 25 BMI, where 23 represents me being pretty lean.

Keep in mind that since this chart is meant as a starting point for all people over a lifetime, know that your target weight may change as you get older. As we age, most of us naturally lose muscle mass, so your ideal BMI may be lower in your 50's than it was in your 30's if you lose muscle mass over the decades.

Don't be that guy who maintains the 200 pounds you weighed in your athletic heyday if that weight shifts from muscle to fat over the years. It is on you to make sure your target weight and BMI line up with a realistic level of leanness - we can't do it for you. Caveats aside, the BMI table is a great starting point to use as a tool to determine a healthy weight for you.

Mark here - I have to add to Henry's comment above. I've known guys over the years that were college athletes and still weigh the same as when they were starting linebackers, therefore think they are are still in great shape. I just want to know where they buy their magic mirrors.

CHAPTER 7:
TOOL BOX

◆ ◆ ◆

Mark here - Now that you have set a target weight you are going to need a few tools and a plan on how to use them for this journey.

***Paper journal or electronic record keeping tools** - I personally use a basic daily weight tracker that is built into iOS. I also use a notes application for notes on food, calories, exercise, progress, etc. Choose whatever method you like, but record everything! After weighing myself each morning, I record the result. Some days I'm happy, some days not. But you must record it!*

***Digital scale** - Buy a digital scale for measuring your weight. Good enough ones can be had for around $30. Measure your weight every morning wearing nothing and after urinating, but before eating or drinking anything. This should give you a consistent measurement. Once you start to lose the pounds, you will experience a true rush when you get on the scale. You might even start weighing yourself at bedtime and guessing what your weight will be in the morning. Many digital scales on the market today also provide you with readings for muscle mass, bone mass, water weight, and more. These measurements are not generally considered to be extremely accurate but should be consistent if you want to geek out and measure your trends beyond pounds.*

***Kitchen scale** - After a while you will get a feel for portion size, but* *in the early days you will need a scale to measure portions. If you eyeball portions, you will almost certainly over estimate portion size.*

Soft tape measure - *The scale measures your pounds, but your waist measurement is also important to track. For men at least, a waist size in the high 30's is a health warning. Too much fat around your organs. Tracking your waist circumference is another way to provide yourself with positive feedback and to visibly measure results. Be careful though, it is hard to measure your waist consistently and accurately. The consensus seems to be to position the tape in a level way around your midsection ½ inch above your belly button. Fun finding - I think you will find that 5 lbs of lost weight equates to 1 inch off your waistline. Try it and see!*

Length of cord - *As an alternative to or instead a tape measure, take a length of non stretchy cord (roughly ¼ diameter) and measure a length that with a knot at each end which is equal to exactly your target waistline goal. Take the time to get this right. When you put this cord around your waist, the knots will not touch until you reach your target. Simple and effective!*

While we are talking about inches, ignore the waist size of your clothing. The real circumference of your waist will almost certainly be higher than your pants size. The smaller sizes might be a marketing ploy. Personally, the pants I buy generally have a waist size 2-3 inches less than my measured waist.

Henry here - I buy pant sizes that fluctuate anywhere from a few inches less than my measured waist to a few inches more. It is a total crapshoot because every brand is different. Don't read into pant sizes across brands. You have more important and accurate indicators you can use.

Mark here - In addition to what the scale says every morning, if you are losing weight, your clothes will get looser, you will feel healthier, and have more energy. Your blood pressure and cholesterol levels may drop and you may be less likely to develop diabetes. Less weight equals less stress on your joints. All good.

All that said, one thing that losing weight doesn't do is change your body shape. We all store fat differently (in different places). Losing weight won't change this, whatever fat you have left will be in the same places and will still be stubborn. Enough exercise performed for long enough (think years) may help.

A note to the ladies - Obviously I am male and write from that perspective. My examples may not always resonate with you. However, the concepts apply equally to men and women. My wife will attest that what I recommend worked for her as well.

Henry here - My father covered the high points: there are really three easy barometers and one harder one to measure your progress. Your weight, your measurements, your clothing size, and how you look. If you really want to see changes in yourself, start taking note of each of them. You probably already do the last two, so let's focus on weight and measurements. Of these two, weight is more important to measure, especially at the beginning of your journey. It is far easier and more painless to stand on a scale than rope a tape-measure around your waist. In addition, if you are significantly overweight, the scale does a fine job in telling you if you are losing fat. Once you become much leaner, the tape measure may become more important, especially if you are trying to build muscle and see your body composition change. For now, let's start with the scale.

As such, step two is like my dad said: get a scale, and start using it. Watch how your weight fluctuates between the morning to evening, and pay attention to what causes it to go up or down. This is your scorecard.

At this point, you have a scorecard, but please, don't be a psycho. No hardcore goals of losing a pound per day. You are to simply be a student of your own body. See what happens. As you try new things, pay attention to if they make you lose or gain weight. You are officially the scientist in charge of your own body and now have ways to quantify it.

You may find that just by tracking your weight, you become motivated and start losing pounds. The old adage that "what is measured, improves" may become your best friend here. Have fun with this and learn as much as you can. This feedback system will become the basis for the rest of your dieting journey.

Now, going back to the "don't be a psycho" point, please do not expect your weight to just drop because you are thinking about it. Don't beat yourself if it goes up, or drops quickly and then goes back to normal levels. That is life. A lot of things you do and eat will have huge effects. Try having a big salty meal with a bunch of carbs and water after - you'll balloon a few pounds the next day, but it will be gone a day after.

You may be waiting for the punchline here: how much weight should you be losing each week? While I'd love to give you a very prescriptive answer - 1.53 pounds per six days - I don't have one. That is because losing weight is a very finicky thing that is different for everyone. Some people, like my dad, lose 28 pounds over two months, and some people go much slower than that.

The danger is that if you lose weight too fast, the process will be miserable, your body will be unhappy and worried that you cut weight too fast, and you will bounce back to your old weight. If you have a lofty goal of rapid weight loss, you are likely to overdo your diet and yo-yo back up.

If you are losing 1-2 pounds per week, that is plenty! Nice work. Even if you are not hitting that every week, don't worry too much. More important than day-to-day fluctuations is weekly and monthly progress. The body is finicky and slow to react, but over time will yield to the environment you put it in. Don't sweat over the short term fluctuations. Be patient and enjoy the ride.

If you are losing more than 1-2 pounds per week, this can be either no big deal, or it can potentially be a future issue. If you are just doing the things recommended in the book, you may have faster weight loss. However, pay attention to how difficult this is psychologically. If you are losing a lot more than 1-2 pounds per week but doing so is a breeze, and you aren't feeling starved and miserable, that is a good sign, and you can carry on your merry way.

If the pounds are flying off but you are miserable, you may be going too fast and should look into slowing down your speed of weight loss. Remember, the long term matters most. If you make things so painful that you immediately relapse into your old ways once you hit your target weight, leading you back to square one, you might as well have never dieted in the first place.

Personally, I function best with changes of about 1 pound per week, which is fast enough to notice the progress, but slow enough that it is gradual on my body and I never feel that hungry.

You'll find the right pace for you. Watch the scale, don't push things, and play the long game. You'll be amazed at what you can accomplish in a year.

CHAPTER 8: WHY ARE YOU DOING THIS?

◆ ◆ ◆

Losing weight is hard. A lot of things will be stacked against your success. Think of this chapter as a pep-talk reminding you just how tough weight loss is and also why this weight loss journey is critical for your current self, future self, and those you care about. You're not doing this just to look pretty in the mirror (though it is a great side effect!). You're doing this to live a fuller life packed with activity long past middle age.

Regardless of whether you are your ideal weight already and are just fighting to maintain it, or if you have a long weight-loss journey ahead of you, know that this is a battle we all face, and the cards are stacked against all of us.

Our bodies cling to higher weights. Once you stay a certain weight for a while, your body gets comfortable with it, creating a weight "set-point" that your body will drift back to if you stop paying attention to your diet. That means if you are overweight now, you either need to change things soon and create a new set point, or accept that you may look the way you do now for the rest of your life.

Actually, it is worse than that. You will probably get heavier if you don't pay careful attention. Those few extra calories and lower activity levels over the years will start to add up into pounds that you won't get rid of. There's no better time than now to fix you set point and make the rest of your life a little easier.

Lowering your set point will be tough, and the heavier you are, the tougher it will be, so you need to start now. I'll save the science for the next few paragraphs, but the scary truth is that the fatter you are, the easier it is to get even fatter. The leaner you are, the easier it is to get and stay leaner. The playing field is not level: it is constantly changing and depending on where you are, can be entirely in your favor or overwhelmingly against you, which can make progress lumpy and inconsistent.

I'm going to summarize the science behind this in the next section, so prepare for things to get more technical.

Mark here - While I believe that no one should be shamed for their choices, I fully believe that the amount a person weighs is a choice, be it an active or a passive choice. I'm hoping that you, our reader, will make a choice to get to and maintain a healthy weight and then make a further choice about the right combination of further weight loss combined with exercise to achieve the desired look and feel for yourself.

Diabetes, Insulin Resistance, and Why Progress is Hard

Henry here - The more body fat you have, the more challenging it becomes for your body to process food, and the less you are filled up by the same amount of food. Just let that sink in for a minute, because the more you think about it, the more you realize the cruelty of it.

The driving force behind this is called insulin resistance by the scientific community. To gain a better understanding of this phenomenon, first one must look into the idea of nutrition and energy levels at the most fundamental level. When you eat, your digestive systems breaks your food into glucose, a simple sugar molecule. This glucose enters your bloodstream in as fast as a few minutes, and your pancreases responds by releasing insulin, a hormone which says to your cells "hey guys, there's sugar in the blood - get some!" A feeding frenzy ensues. In other words, insulin acts as a key, unlocking the doors to glucose in the bloodstream and granting cells access to usable energy.

Normally, the more keys (insulin) there are, the more doors

(cells searching for energy) are unlocked. This dynamic relationship is always in flux. Excess glucose, or high blood sugar, is the result of an insufficient amount of insulin. This excess goes into your liver and is stored as glycogen as your cells are unable to use it. A lack of glucose, or low blood sugar, means there was too much insulin. In a scenario with too much insulin, your cells are opening doors expecting energy on the other side where there is not any, leading to "low energy" symptoms including shakiness, weakness, confusion, and hunger. The remedy? Your body will release glucagon, which tells your liver to release the glycogen into glucose and into your blood, giving your cells the energy they need.

The human body is amazing and knows exactly how much insulin to give to ensure its cells have precisely the energy they need…at least, that is, when it is operating under normal conditions. However, excess body fat can mess up these conditions. As you get fatter, your body's response to insulin decreases, giving you what is called insulin resistance, which is a precursor to diabetes. There is a clear, documented association of higher BMI levels with insulin resistance[6].

Insulin resistance means that when there is sugar in your blood (caused from when you eat), your body releases insulin as normal, but your body doesn't respond to the insulin as well. The cells don't eat as much of the sugar as they should. Extra sugar just hangs out in the bloodstream, and the cells don't get the energy they need. Since your cells don't get the energy they need, you start to feel hungry, even though there is plenty of sugar in your blood already, starting a vicious cycle. The fatter you get, the more this intensifies.

What this means is that when a fatter person eats a bag of donuts, since they are more insulin resistant than a lean person, their body has to release more insulin to get the same effect as a lean person. Not only that, but since their body doesn't respond well to insulin, their body may not have released enough of it into the bloodstream. As a result, more glucose will just sit in the bloodstream rather than being put to use by cells. This may mean they feel less of an energy boost than the lean person and still feel hungry, even after a big meal. This may cause them to eat even more, amplifying the problem.

Let me say that one more time: when you are fatter, food fills you up less.

Not only will the fatter person be less full, but they will have more insulin released. Higher insulin "causes your body to lose muscle while it creates more belly fat, more inflammation, and more oxidative stress. The downstream effects of this—besides an expanding waistline and feeling sleepy all time—are scary. High insulin levels and insulin resistance symptoms are linked to high blood pressure, high cholesterol, high triglycerides, low sex drive, infertility, depression, heart disease, stroke, dementia, cancer—all the common diseases of aging. And the person with insulin resistance will develop one or more of these serious diseases far in advance of their normal time[7]."

This means that the fatter you get, the hungrier you get, the sleepier you get, and the more likely you are to get sick.

If you are creeping up on the scale, stop yourself as soon as possible because it will only get harder. This road can lead to type II Diabetes, which means that your body can't regulate its own blood sugar levels appropriately since it doesn't respond well to insulin. Type II diabetes is partially influenced by genetics, but your weight is the primary (and influenceable) risk factor.

Unfortunately, this means that if you're already fat, you are at a huge disadvantage. Your body does not process foods as well as a lean person, and you will automatically be more tired from your higher residual insulin levels. You will have obstacles, and your body will fight you along the way. This is what happened to me when I "bulked" to 200 pounds: the heavier I got, the hungrier I was, and the easier it was to continue bulking. I've found this to happen even after gaining ten or so pounds: the more weight I gain, the easier it is to keep gaining it.

The good news is that as you get leaner, these symptoms reverse. You'll feel more full and have more energy. You need to get the ball rolling, because it will pick up speed. The leaner you get, the easier it will become! Again, this is something I have repeatedly had happen to myself, and most of my weight cuts have resulted in my accidentally cutting more weight than expected because it became easier as I got lighter and more receptive to insulin.

Fatness and Aging

Now that you're scared to death of insulin resistance, let's go into less alarming but more painful outcomes of being overweight as you get older. I am not even going to address the research about heart attacks and their connection with obesity and even cancer because that is well-documented. Spend a few minutes on google if you want to read more.

Some people have experienced it first-hand, and it can be horrible to see one of your friends die in their fifties. But the thing nobody talks about is just how hard it is to be overweight and live a long and enjoyable life, heart disease aside. Once you become a certain age, your body starts getting weaker. Muscle becomes much harder to build, and slowly declines. I'll let the actual age be something for the scientists to decide, but we can all agree that people start getting weaker in their middle age, which continues until they die.

Imagine that every year, your legs and arms get weaker, but you stay the same weight. Everything gets harder and harder. A simple walk down the block becomes exhausting because of the extra pounds you have to carry with you. That really cuts into your plans of hiking the Appalachian trail, or playing 18 holes of golf every day in retirement. Not only that, but things like chasing and carrying around your grandkids becomes near impossible if you are already carrying dozens of extra pounds of bodyweight.

This weight takes a toll on your joints. Every step means more pressure on already weakening bones. Your odds of breaking something go up with every additional pound you carry. The Johns Hopkins Arthritis Center makes it startlingly clear, saying that "Joint Pain is Strongly Associated with Body Weight" and that "being only 10 pounds overweight increases the force on the knee by 30-60 pounds with each step[8]." The Hopkins center, unsurprisingly, notes that weight loss can help reduce joint pain and prevalence of arthritis.

Even worse than pure joint pain is the biggest danger as you get older: falling. You're probably laughing because worrying about falling down when you're old is likely not high on your list of everyday worries right now. Trust me, add a few decades and you'll realize this is a very real danger, especially if you are carrying extra weight.

Extra pounds widen your center of gravity and mean that once you wobble in one direction, you are more likely to go down. The extra weight means that if you do fall, your impact will be harder. Since you're older, your bones will be more brittle and more likely to break. Finally, the worst part: think about when you fall and put your hand out to catch you. Your hand hits the ground and your muscles contract, trying to absorb the force of your fall and keep the tension off your bones. The weaker your muscles are, the less power you have to cushion your own falls and the more pressure goes into your weakening bones. Therefore, if you age into being both overweight and weak, the odds of each fall leading to a trip to the hospital go up dramatically.

You're probably scoffing right now because you aren't old at all, and have plenty of years left before you have to worry about falling. Maybe you laughed because you are not fat, just a little soft, and the idea of worrying about your center of gravity sounds ridiculous. Ok, fine, maybe you are not that old or that heavy, but in your free time do you play sports? If so, are you nursing an injury? Are you constantly worried about hurting yourself? Do you feel far more tired than you used to when you were younger? Part of this may be simply due to age, but it may also be due to the extra weight you are carrying around.

Don't believe me? Try playing basketball with a ten pound backpack on. You'll notice a difference. Even a few pounds makes an impact.

Now that we've established that being overweight can make things tough, let's explore the flip-side: what it is like to be very lean. Before you go off the deep end here, let me clarify: I'm talking about men having visible abs, somewhere around 10% body fat, and women having an outline of abs, not anorexic or unhealthily low levels of weight. A good benchmark would be similar to, or a little less lean than the models on the cover of Men's Health or Women Health magazines. Any leaner than that is usually temporary, so if you get to this point, congratulations, you've made it to a sustainable peak physique.

For men, any leaner than this would mean having "grainy" body-builder-like muscle definition, and for women it would mean a very chiseled set of abs. These are achievable over short periods of time, but maintaining that level leanness for months at a time may leave you in a state of weakened immune system and, for women, sometimes hampered fertility as menstrual cycles can stop when you achieve a certain level of leanness. So, let's settle for near magazine-cover levels of leanness as our goal, and dig into why society has decided that is so desirable.

While it seems vain and shallow to use getting a sweet set of abs as your benchmark for health goals, I disagree. Many people have argued that the obsession with thinness is a new, media-created idea. Stop right there. Go look at ancient Greek statues. They are rocking abs straight out of a P-90X ad. The ancient Greeks made even their gods jacked. Stop pretending this is a new phenomenon. It isn't.

Carrying less weight means you will be faster, exert yourself less doing the same work, and less likely to tear a muscle or break a bone by putting too much pressure on it. Those sound like pretty good traits if you're trying to survive. Sure, a layer of fat can be beneficial in famines and as a protective buffer against your important organs if you are a gladiator, but for most day-to-day activities, being lighter and leaner gives you the edge. Besides, the last time I checked, famines are becoming rarer and rarer, and armed sword combat jobs are quite hard to find these days.

Abs are literally a sign that you are a healthy and strong person. Stop demonizing them and realize that if you get and maintain them, you will be in a state of higher performance in all aspects of your life. They also come with a lot of fun side-effects. The attractive chiseled jaw-lines every guy wants? They are much more visible with less fat around your face. Those skinny arms girls always want to have? Again, less body fat. Take a look at some before and after weight-loss photos of people. In most cases, their faces become more conventionally attractive.

If you are frustrated with society's obsession on skinniness, I challenge you to see it differently by thinking of your future partner. If you are married, think of your current partner. Let's make three assumptions:

First, let's assume that someone is overweight, they are likely to continue to be overweight. Let's say they have a 71% chance of remaining overweight, and a 29% chance of losing weight. These are not random numbers - in 2016, 71% of Americans were overweight[9].

Second, let's assume that people lose their muscle mass as they get older.

Third, let's assume that you and your partner either have children already, or plan to have children.

Now, with these three assumptions, imagine you are choosing between two marriage partners who are exactly the same height, with the same personality, job, and friend circle. You are very close to both of them and have great chemistry with both. They have similar families and you get along with both swimmingly. You love everything about both potential partners. The only difference between them is that one is a few pounds overweight and one is lean. You are attracted to both and don't prefer one over the other. It seems that both are great choices.

Hang on. Remember the assumptions we made. If you choose the overweight partner, the odds are that they will stay overweight. As they age, they, just like the other partner, will also lose muscle mass and mobility. With every passing decade, this will intensify and affect the overweight partner more. By the time you have children, your partner will be slower, making it tough to keep up with them. Once grandkids come around, forget it - your partner may barely be able to walk, let alone run. Not to mention all the other health conditions that come with excess weight. You chose an option that seemed to matter little at the time, but amplified over the years.

Now, this is all hypothetical, so it may not happen this way, but shows that there may actually be a biological rationale behind the attractiveness of skinny people. They simply are expected to have longer, healthier, more mobile lives. It is hard to pass up on that. So before you rail against the media for focusing more on skinny people, remember, there may be a kernel of truth in there.

If you are already overweight or have a partner who is, consider this a wakeup call to take action before it is too late. The consequences will come slowly and sneak up on you, but they will manifest themselves.

I admit that there is a whole separate set of problems with the media's tendency to photoshop models and depict unrealistic expectations. That is an important issue worthy of its own book that I will not get into. My point is simply that the preference for leanness is not inherently immoral or wrong.

Before you throw the book across the room with dozens of holes in my argument, I will also admit that being lean does not always mean you are healthy. Not at all. You can be super lean and a chainsmoker but about to get lung cancer. However, if you took a lean chainsmoker and an obese one, everything else equal, in almost all cases, the obese one would have more health issues and a harder everyday life. Similarly, being overweight does not mean you are automatically less attractive. However, in many instances, losing weight (to a healthy extent - not getting leaner than our "magazine-cover" standard) will increase your attractiveness in addition to health.

The next time some smug friend pooh-poohs you for trying to get in better shape, know that doing this will bring you decades of happier, more action-packed life. The fruits of your labor may not manifest themselves for months, or even years, but they will make an impact. This journey is worth the pain and effort. Stick with it. You are building a foundation for the rest of your life.

CHAPTER 9: START WITH SODA

◆ ◆ ◆

Ok, the pep talk is over. Now you know why you're doing this, and you have your basic set of tools to measure your progress. Let's start making some lifestyle changes.

Your first step may be your easiest: stop consuming sugary drinks. They are the fastest way in the universe to gain fat. They give you calories without filling you up. In this chapter, "soda" will represent all sugary drinks, not just carbonated drinks specifically. This means all the good stuff: carbonated drinks, fruit juice, punch, sports drinks, you name it.

Here's the confusing part: sugary drinks don't have a lot of calories themselves. A standard 12 ounce can of soda only has around 150 calories. Despite that, sugary drinks negatively impact your body composition and the rest of your diet, making everything else harder. You may even find yourself getting hungrier after drinking them. Sugary drinks have been found to be so unhealthy that New York City tried to ban selling soda drinks above a certain size.

Remember everything in the last chapter about insulin resistance? Sugary drinks can cause and worsen it, since they are pure sugar that goes directly into your bloodstream. In contrast, more complex carbohydrates like grains and potatoes at least have to be broken down first by the body, making them digest slower and filling you up as your stomach stays full longer since it has more work to do. There is no better way to mess up your body's insulin processing capabilities described in the last chapter than guzzling soda.

If you drink a lot of sugary drinks now, this won't be easy, because sugar is addictive. Soda is "cool" and delicious and water just doesn't compare. Nobody is disagreeing with that. But if you keep drinking sugary drinks, the rest of your diet will be a lot less effective. It is probably not worth even trying to eat healthy and have more veggies if you're still sabotaging yourself with sugary drinks, so save yourself the heartache and don't bother dieting if you are still going to pour gallons of sugar down your throat. So make it happen, or decide that you are ok with not being any leaner than you are now. Your choice.

This doesn't mean you can't ever eat anything sweet again. Just eat your calories, don't drink them. Forget the apple juice - have the full apple. You will give up from exhaustion before you get too fat from eating fresh fruit, so use that to satiate your sweet tooth.

Some people demonize fruits because of their sugar content. While fruits do have sugar, they also have fiber that fills you up and they are not very calorically dense. They also require chewing, slowing you down. Fruit juice just takes the sugar and water, removing the fiber and making it nutritionally about the same as soda.

A final word of warning: beware of "healthy" sugary drinks. Most of these are hidden within fruity drinks that advertise how many vitamins and servings of fruit they contain. Before you chug these, take a look at the nutrition facts, and compare them to a canned soda. I'm sorry for your loss when you realize that the Coca-Cola has less sugar.

The other sad news is that most of the smoothie-type drinks that are actually good for you and don't have that much sugar in them usually taste like eating sticks. There are no freebies in the sweet drinks territory.

To keep things simple for yourself, I'd suggest steering clear of diet soda and milk until you've reached your goal weight. At that point, experiment with them, but until then you'll likely make faster progress if you stay away altogether. With regards to diet soda specifically, scientists are still looking into it, but some believe that it spikes your blood sugar just like normal soda and leads to fat gain[10]. I choose to play it safe and treat diet soda just like normal soda.

Mark here - The best endorsement I can give to Henry's no soda recommendation is that I stopped drinking soda altogether in 2001. You will lose weight without it.

So Long, Soda!

I said before I don't like to ban foods, but I think soda is different because it is unparalleled in its ability to ruin your physique. Duh - we knew that, but knowing doesn't matter if we keep drinking it. Let's build an anti-soda system to not only help you not drink soda, but also to limit the damage if you aren't ready to ban it altogether. This is where we really start applying behavioral finance to dieting. Our system will focus on two things: lowering your cravings for it, and raising the hurdle to get it.

Lowering Cravings

Here's a scary thought: when you are craving soda, your body may actually need something else but not understand what it really needs. Odds are that you are just in need of some water, or nutrients from normal food. To fight this, next time you want a soda, drink a big glass or two of water, and see if your craving remains. Wait a few minutes and then assess if you still want soda. You may have just been thirsty, and no longer want a soda after having enough water.

If you still want a soda after the water, plan to have it after your next meal. Not just after, but wait twenty or so minutes after you finish eating for your body to process how satiated it is. Hopefully, your craving was just your body telling you that it was hungry, and passes once you eat.

If, after the big glass(es) of water and the meal, you still want a soda, it's time to move to the next step: have another serving of veggies and gulp another glass of water. You want to fill up your stomach as much as you possibly can without actually adding extra calories so that you are so full that the thought of soda is sickening.

If you're still in need of the soda, or can't resist the thought of something sweet, go for some fruit. A single can of soda, which you can gulp down in a few seconds, has approximately 150 calories. A large apple has around 115 calories. Good luck eating the apple as fast as you can chug a soda. Similarly, most berries have very few calories for the amount of chewing you need to do to eat them.

Adding the fruit in may seem counterintuitive because it does provide additional calories. Yet if it quenches your need for something sweet and you begin to use it as your sugary drink replacement, your cravings may start to change from sugary drink cravings to fruit cravings. This sounds crazy, but it happens as your stomach bacteria composition changes based on what you eat. In simple terms, when you eat something, your stomach is more likely to want you to eat that thing again, so shifting to whole fruit increases your chances of eating more fruit instead of drinking sugary drinks.

Now, if after you've already had a few glasses of water, a full meal, an extra serving of vegetables, and a piece of fruit, you still crave soda - wow, you must really want it! By now, you should be so full that you are just about ready to pop. This is exactly what you want. At this point, it should take significantly less willpower to resist the soda craving, which is what we wanted in the first place. If you can resist your soda craving by now, congratulations! If not, keep reading.

Raising the Soda Hurdle

You've had a long journey to get here, and thrown many obstacles at your stomach to stop it on its sugary quest, but have not yet succeeded. Fear not, there is more you can do! You need to make actually getting this soda that you still want so difficult that it is almost not worth the effort, and once you get it, you need to drink as little of it as possible.

The easiest way to make it hard to get is to never buy it at the grocery store. If you have soda sitting around in your fridge, you have already lost. Especially if it is in a 2 liter bottle that you can just pour a little bit into a glass, you're a goner because a bottle like that makes it so easy to just have a sip here and there, accidentally drinking large quantities throughout the day. Cans help because they delineate by serving size, but they are not much better - if they are just a simple walk away in your fridge, you may still be doomed to failure.

If you are going to have a sugary drink, it should be a journey to get. If you are going to have it, only purchase single-serving containers, ideally at a vending machine or convenience store, and get the smallest size you can. Adding the additional hurdle to achieving sugary drinks will reduce the odds of you actually having any. Laziness often wins the day, so make it work for you, instead of against you!

Now, once you've made the journey to get the soda, it doesn't end here. You don't just get to gulp it down in the convenience store like an animal. You're more sophisticated than that, so you're going to have to wait until you get home. Once you get there, find a shot glass and a comfy chair. Fill up the shot glass with your soda and get comfy in the chair. Now, finally, take a sip of the soda and savor it. Drink it slowly so you can truly enjoy the flavor. The rest of the can is all yours, but only if you drink it shot glass by shot glass, and only when you're sitting in the comfy chair.

The second you stop enjoying the soda, or get tired of getting up to refill your shot glass, pour what's left down the sink. At that point, you're not drinking for enjoyment anymore, so it isn't worth having any. You're done and should get rid of the remaining soda as fast as possible. Do not leave yourself vulnerable to future temptations.

By splitting the soda up into shot glass servings, you change it from a single serving (one can) to approximately 8 (a standard 12 ounce can is comprised of 8 1.5 ounce shot glasses). It is a lot harder to go back for eighths than it is to have one serving. By filling your stomach first and drinking it slowly, you blunted your body's insulin response, making the soda marginally less fattening.

Hopefully this whole ordeal is so much work that you decide having sugary drinks is not worth the trouble. Over time, your body will psychologically associate soda with hassle rather than pure bliss, and you will want it less. You have re-programmed yourself for a healthier future. Congratulations!

These same ideas that you used with soda can apply to any kind of food that you are trying to eat less of. The concept of pre-eating and raising the barriers to entry will help you in any scenario, so try this out with anything else you're trying to reduce in your life.

Soda Summed Up

To recap, sugary drinks of all forms are bad for you and will derail your fitness progress faster than almost any normal food. You should avoid them altogether if you can. If you just have to have something sweet, eat fruit so you will have less total calories and fill up your stomach with solid fibrous contents. If you can't stand to live without sugary drinks, before you have any, try making it as hard as possible to have by doing the steps we outlined above:

Drink lots of water first. Eat a full meal. Eat another serving of veggies and glass of water. Have a piece of fruit. If you still want the sugary drink, go to the store and buy a single can. Drink it out of a shot glass, with the can across the room so you have to fill up between glasses. Throw the rest of the can out the second you aren't enjoying it anymore.

Good luck!

CHAPTER 10: SLEEP YOURSELF SKINNY

◆ ◆ ◆

Now I know you're all fired up after realizing that you are in worse shape than you thought and getting motivated by realizing that your goal for leanness will make your life healthier and longer, but take a deep breath. Relax. Your second step towards that healthier and longer life will be a lot less work than you thought. I promised we'd start light and work to the harder stuff if the easy stuff doesn't produce results, so it doesn't get any easier than this:

You need to sleep more.

You're probably thinking that you sleep as much as you can, or that your sleep schedule is just fine. Maybe you're right, but if you're not, you are missing a lot of benefits. It is worth spending some time investigating. Sleep is crucial, and if you are not getting it right, you might be dramatically slowing down both your dieting progress and your overall life happiness. This chapter will outline why sleep is important, and suggest some ways to help you get more of it. If, after reading this, you are still having trouble sleeping, you should consider talking to your doctor. For some people, trouble sleeping is the sign of a bigger problem that needs to be addressed.

Sleep is truly a magical thing, and if you deprive yourself of it, your mental performance declines. Staying up for long periods puts your mind in a state of unawareness that is equivalent to being drunk[11]. Along with that, your willpower weakens and you become more likely to make poor eating choices. In addition to the willpower, lack of sleep can make you moody and generally unhappy.

Maybe you knew that, but did you know that less sleep messes up your body's hormones in a way that makes you hungrier too?

Studies have found that sleep deprivation increases hunger and appetite, especially for high carbohydrate foods[12]. Scientists find that even a week of sleep deprivation leads to a pre-diabetic state even in healthy subjects[13]. Lack of sleep raises your cortisol (stress hormone), lowers your leptin (fullness hormone), and raises your ghrelin (hunger hormone)[14].

Some people have even said that the rise in obesity rates over the past few decades has been correlated with a decline in average sleep levels[15]. Now hopefully you're listening.

The good news is that sleep is wonderful for the body. It allows your body to repair itself, to process things you learned during the day and transfer them to long-term memory, and helps your immune system stay strong. Especially if you are exercising, sleep is key to helping your body recover.

More than that, sleeping accomplishes a wonderfully practical thing: when you're asleep, you can't be eating.

Mark here - The first time I ever heard this was from a college roommate who swore by the idea that you can't eat while you sleeping.

Henry here - I know, that sounds really stupid. Obviously you can't eat when you are asleep. But think about it: when you have a very early day or a long day, you will usually eat a bit more. You'll have that 5am breakfast before you get going, or that 11pm snack before bed. Had you just been asleep that time, you wouldn't have eaten. I see this firsthand all the time: on weekends, when I sleep more, I miss meals sometimes purely by sleeping through them, and usually end up losing weight over the weekend. So, to clarify, you should be sleeping more for four reasons:

First, if you don't sleep, you will be tired and your willpower will be lower, so you'll make bad eating decisions.

Second, Lack of sleep can make you more likely to get sick, in addition to generally grouchy and unhappy.

Third, if you don't sleep enough, your hormones will make you hungrier and you will crave unhealthy foods.

Fourth, If you do sleep enough, you may sleep through meals and snack less simply because you are not awake to do so.

I am not saying you need to sleep 12 hours per night. I just ask that you pay attention to how much you are sleeping, and try to improve either the quality or the quantity.

A lot of people think that sleep is something that "just happens" to them, and claim that if that wasn't the case, they wouldn't fall asleep naturally when they are tired. That misses the point. Everyone passes out due to exhaustion at some point, but that doesn't mean they are getting enough rest. Good, quality sleep actually requires you getting a lot of variables just right. There are people whose entire jobs are focused on helping people get better sleep, and maybe you need to see them at some point, but before you do, I want to share some things to look into before you spend the extra time and money.

Many of us have probably played the early morning "I'll get to bed early the night before" game. It goes like this:

You usually go to bed around 11, but have a super early morning the next day, and rush to get to bed early. You workout at 7 instead of 8 that night, hurry to finish your post-workout meal, and rush through your chores to get everything done early. At 8:59, you fall onto your pillow, triumphant at how early you managed to get there and ecstatic about how well-rested you'll be tomorrow.

You stare at the ceiling with a huge grin on your face, waiting to blissfully fall asleep. Then your leg starts itching and you remember that you forgot to check something. You get up and fix that thing, then come back to bed. Then you are a little too warm, so you turn the air conditioning down. Then you can't get comfortable, and toss and turn. You start thinking about a memory from years ago, wondering what happened to Roger from high school. You decide you have to look him up on Facebook, and then spend 20 minutes scrolling through his photos. After that, you're determined to get back to sleep.

The cycle repeats. You just can't relax. You start to realize it is getting late and you get stressed. Your heart rate goes up and you get mad at yourself for not being able to calm down and fall asleep. You consider getting a therapist to talk to your problems with. Finally, around 11, you fall asleep at your normal time and wake up tired the next morning. The cycle repeats ad infinitum.

Forget the therapist. Your body is tricking the heck out of you. It is likely that you aren't really that stressed out, but are being fooled by your hormones and internal clock. If those are out of whack, you will feel restless and have more energy around bedtime. You may only notice that you can't shut your brain down and keep coming up with all sorts of interesting thoughts, rather than having physical energy. Regardless, the outcome is the same: you can't get to sleep. Don't worry about this being some underlying mental issue. It may just be that you are overlooking some important variables to your sleep. Let's dig into the most important factors.

Timing

Timing is a monster that will make-or-break your sleep schedule. Your body thrives on regularity and if you can manage to go to bed at the same time every day, you'll fall asleep like clockwork. That is why you always hear doctors preach a consistent bedtime.

Going to bed at the same time is the holy grail, but let's be honest: you aren't a monk. You have friends, maybe children, hobbies, and work to do. You may not be able to get to bed at the same time every night. What you will find is that you can usually stay up a few hours later without much difficulty, but once you do, you push your set bedtime later by those few hours and it becomes tough to reset.

For example, let's say you normally go to bed at 9. One day, you stay up till 11 instead and sleep in 2 hours later than normal. The next day, you try to go to bed at 9 again, only to find that you can't fall asleep until 11. You seem doomed in this cycle of increasingly later bedtimes, as the body loves to reset to a later bedtime but won't obey you when you want to go the other way and fall sleep earlier.

There are only two workarounds for this that I've had consistent luck with: get up early the next day, making your body super tired and forcing it to crash at 9 the next day like you want, or take melatonin to help reset your bedtime earlier.

I was scared of taking anything for years because I try to avoid pills and drugs when I can, but I admit that melatonin has been life-changing for me. For entire decades of my life, I spent every Sunday night lying in bed praying that I'd fall asleep and not be exhausted the next morning, but unable to since I'd stayed up late on Saturday and slept in on Sunday. I could never fall asleep when I wanted to. In college, I had the realization that I had never beaten the cycle, and decided I would just stop pretending I'd fall asleep early, and planned to stay up anyway.

The outcome on Monday was the same regardless of when I tried to fall asleep: I was exhausted and reset to an earlier bedtime Monday night. However, at least if I stayed up on Sunday night I could at least get a few more hours of productivity or fun back.

Recently, I took the plunge to melatonin because it is a natural hormone your body produces, and started taking 5 mg on nights when I'm trying to get to bed earlier than the previous night. I'm happy to report that it has broken the cycle, and I can fall asleep whenever I want to now.

Before you get too ahead of yourself, getting your timing right or taking some melatonin before bed does not negate the need to get the other variables right. It may be the most important factor, but if you are messing the next few pieces of the puzzle, you still won't have a great night's sleep.

In fact, as of the writing of this book, melatonin is slightly controversial. While there is evidence (including first-hand from myself) that it can be very helpful to help you fall asleep, some studies have found it to be more of a placebo effect than anything else[16]. Recommended doses range from two tenths of a milligram to five milligrams[17], and there can be side effects from taking large doses. Melatonin may interact with other medications you are taking, and its long term side effects are still being studied and currently unknown. With all this in mind, I suggest you talk to your doctor about melatonin before taking any, and if you do end up using it, do so sparingly.

Melatonin or not, the other variables described below are crucial for quality sleep.

Light

I spent 8 years of my childhood in Singapore, which is a 19-21 hour flight from Newark airport, depending on wind conditions. Twice per year, my family and I would make the trip back to visit either my Mom's parents in Atlanta, or my Dad's parents in New Mexico. Adding in layovers and commute time to and from the airports, the journey usually took about 30 hours door-to-door. For most of this time, we would have no idea either where in the world we were, or what day it was. When we finally made it to our destination, we would immediately crash in our beds. Yet we always woke up at weird times. I distinctly remember the four of us, jet-lagged and playing the board game "Life" in my grandmother's kitchen at 3am.

To get over the jet-lag, the name of the game was always trying to stay up through the whole day without naps. If you could make it to a normal bedtime for a few days in a row, you could reset your internal clock enough to be adjusted to the new timezone. Every single year, I was the first person to get adjusted. Staying up was hard for everyone, but I was almost always the exception who could make it past dinner. We could all usually get through the afternoon as long as we went outside, stayed moving, and got lots of sunlight, but the rest of my family rarely made it past dinner.

Why was I the only one doing it?

It wasn't a willpower thing. I was doing something that nobody else was: playing videogames. I always had a video game console or computer nearby that I would jam away at. This was before devices had "night-shift mode", so my eyes were being flooded nonstop with the eerie electric blue glow of my screens. I'd play for hours, effortlessly staying awake while everyone else crashed.

Mark here - I can't resist throwing in a parenting comment related to Henry's mention of video game play. In our early days in Singapore we lived in a large one level condo with marble floors throughout. Henry didn't care at all about health, fitness, or nutrition back then, but he sure cared about playing video games. He had an office-type chair with wheels at his gaming station and he would ride that chair all over the condo as if he couldn't walk. He mostly did it to annoy me - it worked.

Henry here again - It's funny, I never did the chair thing to bug my dad. It was just such an efficient system to use the same chair everywhere rather than having to walk around, or change chairs to eat dinner. I felt like the single chair made my life easier and better. While I now realize that having multiple chairs is not what is making people's lives too complex, the idea of simplifying life with a system has stuck with me, and that is what this book aims to do.

Back to the video games. We couldn't figure it out at the time, but years later I discovered a program called F.lux and things started to click.

The thesis behind F.lux is that your brain thinks that the blue light emitted from TV, computer, and phone screens is sunlight, and so when you look at screens at night, your body is fooled into thinking that it is daytime and releases hormones that keep you awake. Cue the sleepless nights and trouble falling asleep. Sounds sketchy, huh? Spend some time on the F.lux website[18]. They have plenty of academic studies showing that the blue light effect is very real, and I now understand that it is what allowed me to keep myself up as late as I wanted in those jetlagged international travel days.

Where this takes us is that light can really screw up your sleep.

I trust that nobody is trying to sleep with their lights on, so let's focus on the more subtle fixes. If you don't have dark curtains in your room, consider getting some. Your best sleep will be in absolute darkness. Try to dim your lights near bedtime and to minimize light when you are sleeping as much as possible. As far as electronics, try to not use them before bed, or if you absolutely must, get an app like F.lux to make your screen orange rather than blue. I've found that I can fall asleep about 2 hours after seeing blue light. For those Apple device users, there is a setting called nightshift mode that does the same thing as F.lux.

We are now very lucky that things like nightshift mode and F.lux exist and we don't have to do what I did years ago: wear orange sunglasses after dark to earn the nickname "Cyclops" from my friends.

Light may be your enemy when you are trying to fall asleep, but it is your best friend when you are trying to wake up and stay awake. It is as simple as turning the lights on and opening the curtains to help wake yourself up. If you need to stay up for something, skip the book and blast the television. Happy lighting!

Food, Drink and Exercise

The next mistake a lot of people make before going to sleep is eating, drinking, or exercising close to bedtime. Don't do it - it will just get your body riled up. The exact times for everyone will vary, but I've found that for me, about 2 hours before bed is the magic number. It is also worth looking into your caffeine consumption - even coffee in the early afternoon might be messing up your sleep. Everyone handles caffeine differently and has their own tolerance for it, but it can really mess you up at night if you aren't careful.

Also, for those chocolate lovers out there, beware that cocoa has modest amounts of caffeine in it, so if you're crushing that

Special Dark before bed, or having items with extra cocoa powder in them, it might keep you up. I learned this the hard way after making chocolate casein protein brownies with extra cocoa power and having many sleepless nights.

The flip side of this is that food, drink, and exercise will help you wake up. I've had great results by putting my alarm across the room so I have to walk to turn it off. I usually find that the walk wakes me up and dramatically reduces the odds of me hitting snooze.

Temperature

The final piece of being able to sleep well is making sure your body temperature isn't too high or too low. 68 degrees Fahrenheit (20 degrees celsius) is a number usually thrown around, but try experimenting and see what works for you. A lot of the trouble people run into is from their body temperature being too high, which can be a side-effect of it still being pumped up from exercise, or heating up while digesting food or drink. One way, outside of what we've already talked about, of getting your body temperature down before bed is taking a hot shower before bed. The heat will nudge your body to cool itself down, and counterintuitively, your body temperature will drop afterwards, allowing you to get a good night's sleep.

Tying it all Together

Hopefully what I've shared with you so far about getting better sleep has been helpful. If not, then maybe a sleep therapist is the solution. For a simpler solution, spend some time reading on sleep.org, a website by the National Sleep Foundation focused on the positive benefits of sleep health, which has a wealth of content. More than likely you know how to sleep enough now, but are just not doing it. Execution is really important. I know - you're busy - just like everyone else. But you don't have to be healthier, and you don't have to be your goal weight: it is a choice.

If you want it that bad, find a way to get enough sleep. Maybe you are one of those lucky people that functions well on 6 hours of sleep, but you might just be lying to yourself. Try getting 8 hours for a few weeks. See if anything else in your life changes. You might just be surprised.

CHAPTER 11: ONE STEP AT A TIME

◆ ◆ ◆

When I was in college, every single time I came home to my parents' house between semesters, I would gain two to four pounds over the week or two. As someone who pays a lot of attention to my weight, I was alarmed because it didn't make any sense. It would happen even when I ate significantly less food than I did at school. For a while, I was convinced that my parents were lacing the food they cooked with extra butter, or that it was just something in the air in Florida where they lived.

One day everything clicked when of my classmates complained that all the buildings on campus were so far away from each other. The wheels started turning in my head. My apartment was a mile away from campus, and I walked both ways. Campus itself was maybe a half mile across, and I spent the entire day criss-crossing it to get to different classes and activities. The whole time I was hoofing around with a heavy backpack, racking up a lot of steps.

Meanwhile, at home in Florida, we drove everywhere we went. Sometimes I would take a walk with my parents around the neighborhood, but we only went a half mile or so. In contrast to the four or more miles I probably did every day at school with a heavy bag on my back, I was essentially sedentary when I was at home. I think that caused my weight gain when I came home, and the subsequent loss when I returned to school.

No fancy supplements, no clever diets, just good old fashioned walking.

Some things are as old as dirt for a reason. Walking as a form of exercise is one of them. Sadly, it is often overlooked for its sexier cousin, running. Everyone and their mother decides that when they are serious about losing weight, they are going to lace up their Nikes and go on eight mile runs until one day they look in the mirror and realize they look exactly like the model in the Nike ads.

Then they actually go running, and it sucks. Their feet hurt. They get blisters. Their shins and knees ache. But they know it is just a matter of pushing through, because no pain no gain. Then, they finally finish their run, dizzy from exhaustion, and pat themselves on the back for a job well done.

The next morning, they wake up and attempt to lift their legs off the bed. They find aching pain in every direction. For the first time in their life, they realize their legs are not working, and have to be physically lifted to get them out of bed. They step onto the floor, quivering like a baby lamb walking for the first time. A huge grin of victory lights their face, as they are so proud to be more sore than they ever have been in their entire life. They hobble over to their new running shoes, lace up, and go for another run.

This ends three ways:

Option one: They become a jogger, and start running marathons. They make friends with other runners and begin running everywhere.

Option two: They keep running, ignoring the fact that they are sore almost every time they go, and have increasingly noticeable aches and pains in their joints. One day they hear a pop and find out they sprained something and need to stop running for a few weeks while it heals. They cry to the heavens, asking why they were punished and how they will ever be fit without being able to run.

Option three: They realize that they dread running and all the hardship associated with it. One day they wake up and refuse to ever run again. They throw away their running shoes and never look back.

I'll let you decide which ending your running fairytale takes, but I will take a guess that even if you start with option one, over time, you either hurt yourself - option two - or end up burning yourself out - option three.

To be clear, running isn't bad. It is a lot of fun. There is a wonderful sense of freedom you can only get by running out of the house with no plans and nothing but open road in front of you. There is a magical sense of accomplishment from being entirely winded and proud of beating a personal record.

Yet running isn't necessary for weight loss. In fact, I'd argue that from a multi-decade perspective, walking trounces it in terms of weight loss effectiveness.

Let's start with some stats. The table below outlines calories burned by 30 minutes of walking at a normal, 3 miles per hour pace, depending on your weight, compared to 30 minutes of running at a normal, 6 miles per hour pace[19].

Weight	Calories burned from 30 minutes walking (1.5 miles walked)	Calories burned from 30 minutes running (3 miles ran)
100	83	233
150	125	350
200	167	467
250	208	583

You probably looked at this table and thought "gee, I really should be running!" But hang on. There's more to it. What if you walk a little faster?

Weight	Calories burned from 30 minutes walking (1.75 miles walked)	Calories burned from 30 minutes walking (2 miles walked)
100	102	119
150	154	179
200	205	238
250	256	298

Two trends are clear.

First, the heavier you are, the more calories you burn, no

matter what you do. A 250 pound person burns about as many calories in 30 minutes of walking as a 100 pound person does in 30 minutes of running.

This means that the heavier you are, the less you actually need to run. Your body has a lot of work to do just to carry the weight, so keep walking until you need to run. When you're 100 pounds, you may have to start running, but for now, enjoy the luxury of not needing to!

Second, the faster you move, the more calories you burn. This should not be a surprise to anyone, but keep in mind that walking can move the needle more than you might think, especially at higher paces. You may read this and then decide that you should do all-out sprints. On a per-minute basis, you are correct, but you're missing the big picture: the sustainability and enjoyment of the activity.

Let's say you are 150 pounds, and you can run three times per week, for 30 minutes each session, for a total of 90 minutes of total exercise. That is all the time you have to fit in your schedule.

That gets you 350 calories per 30 minute session, so 350 times 3 is 1,050 calories per week burned. Alternatively, you can accomplish this through walking 4 hours and 12 minutes per week. This could be accomplished through a single 36 minute walk every day. Assuming that is broken into a round-trip journey, that means walking to and from somewhere that is approximately 18 minutes.

One of these activities - the walk - is something you can do with anyone of any age accompanying you, where you can chat and have a nice time and not be soaked in sweat afterwards.

The other one - the run - is generally a solitary activity where you stress about how fast you are going and how sore you are afterwards.

Another variable not being considered is cleanup time. Let's say you weigh 150 pounds and have 3 miles per day of distance you need to cover. On one hand, you can walk it at a 3 mile per hour pace and get it done in an hour of walking. On the other hand, you can run it at a 6 mile per hour pace and get it done in a half hour of running. Running burns 350 calories instead of 250 (doubling the 125 in our previous table), and takes half the time.

40% more calories burned and half the time is a very tempting offer. But this takes out the opportunity cost of the preparation for the running. You have to get your running outfit and shoes on. You have to find that right playlist. You have to stretch for a few minutes. Then when you finish, you have to shower and clean up and eat that thing you always eat after you run. After accounting for all those bells and whistles, the all-in time for the run looks a lot closer to an hour. The friction that all this extra time adds raises the barrier to entry to consistently running, decreasing the odds that you will be able to do it for multiple decades through all of life's surprises and changes.

With the walk, all you do is get your shoes on, walk, and carry on with your day. You even have time (and more importantly, breath) to make phone calls and catch up with friends and family.

Following this purely mathematical logic, if you want a run to be worth it, you better run fast and long enough to make it worth the prep and cooldown time. If it isn't worth the time, bust out those walking shoes!

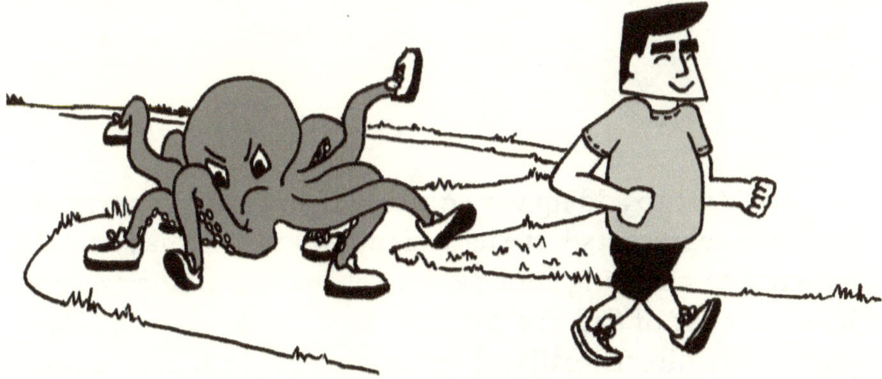

You may be still stewing over the fact that running does burn more calories per mile than walking, and not ready to become a walker. Let's think about this differently. Still assuming you weigh 150 pounds, let's imagine two scenarios.

In the first scenario, you run 3 miles per day at a 6 mile per hour pace, seven days per week. This means 30 minutes of running every day. I imagine it will be hard to actually do this without missing a day, but let's assume that if you miss a day or two, you'll run longer the next day, so you still hit 21 miles per week. You exercise a total of 3.5 hours per week.

In the second scenario, you also travel 3 miles per day, seven days per week, but it is at a 3 miles per hour walking pace. This is an hour of total exercise per day, but as pointed out before, likely takes about the same time as the running per day due to prep time. You exercise a total of 7 hours per week.

Let's imagine that you are able to do both of these routines for an entire year, or five years, or even ten. Let's also play along with the commonly-cited idea that a pound of body fat requires about 3,500 calories of a deficit to burn[20]. Now, what happened over the 1, 5, and 10 year periods of your consistent exercise?

Weight	Calories Burned		Pounds	
	Walking	Running	Walking	Running
Per day	250	350	0.1	0.1
Per week	1,750	2,450	0.5	0.7
Per month	7,000	9,800	2.0	2.8
Per year	91,000	127,400	26.0	36.4
Per 5 years	455,000	637,000	130.0	182.0
Per decade	910,000	1,274,000	260.0	364.0

Things start to add up very quickly if you can be consistent. This table represents just the weight you might theoretically lose without changing your diet, if you just add in the exercise. There are a lot of flaws to simplifying it all down to a calorie number, but directionally, there is a lot of truth here. Even if this number in this table is twice as large as it should be, it would still mean that walking every day is a 13 pound difference over a year.

A better way to think about it would be not just weight you lose by walking, but weight you don't gain because you burn it off from walking. That means you can eat more and still weigh the same! Sounds pretty great to me.

Go back to the table and think about how much of an impact this can have over the course of a lifetime. These amounts of pounds are the difference between losing your mobility from your weight and leading a healthy life.

If you are like many people, you see the 250 calorie figure and scoff, remembering the time the elliptical machine told you about the 1,100 calories you burned that day at the gym and knowing that walking is for suckers. You're thinking about it wrong. Change your benchmark. Think about it in reverse. Imagine if you ate a Snickers bar every day. What would happen? Would you get fat?

A standard 1.56 ounce candy bar has around 200 calories, so walking an hour per day is like removing an entire candy bar from your daily caloric intake. Not so insignificant now, huh?

Build Activity into Your Daily Life

Walking is great, but how do we make it stick?

The simplest solution to walk more is to sell your car and move to a city. You'll be forced to walk, bike, or take public transportation, and can almost guarantee a huge boost to your activity. The great thing about most cities is that while you can have a car, it is often such a hassle to deal with finding and paying for parking where you live that it is often not worth having one. The roads are often so congested that it is only marginally faster to drive somewhere than to walk. The trains or buses are usually much cheaper and at times faster than driving yourself or taking a taxi.

In a city, the path of least resistance leads you to walking most of the time, or at the very least, walking to the train station or bus stop. By default, this makes it much harder to be overweight in a city. Using our tables from earlier in this chapter, even a short 10 minute walk every day could mean around 4 pounds burned every year, so your city-version is 40 pounds better off after a decade of living there. Not only that, but in cities, food generally costs more and restaurants serve smaller portions, so living in one may naturally cause you to eat less.

Yes, you can do this, even in cold or wet places. Get rain gear. Get snow gear. In the summer, commute early in the day before it is blazingly hot. It has been done by humans for centuries, and you can do it too.

If you have decided you can't or will not move to the city, you will have to do a bit more planning. Don't feel bad: there are plenty of valid reasons to not live in a city, and there are other ways to get your walking in. The lowest-hanging fruit is your commute. How much time per day do you spend in a car, train, or bus, sitting and waiting to get to work?

Imagine if you had that commuting time back. What would you do with it? Of course, I want you to say "exercise!" but even if you have other things to do, those are probably much better for you than commuting. Seriously, almost anything else you could think of would be less stressful or more fun than traveling to your job, and the psychological benefit of taking that stress away might have more of an impact on your health than you think.

Maybe moving to the city isn't feasible, but are you able to move to within a mile and a half of your job? If so, suddenly your commute to and from work, which you have to do anyway, becomes your 250 calories of exercise and you never have to think about it again.

This is the ideal: finding a way to make walking a habit that you automatically do every day. If you can do that, you will have all these extra calories that you can either just burn off to lose weight or you can now eat more and maintain your current weight. Enjoy!

Sadly, a lot of the United States is either hard or actually impossible to walk across. Sidewalks are a luxury that doesn't always exist. While this is an obstacle, it is changing ever so slowly as cities recognize the need for walking and rebuild themselves to be more walkable. Hopefully this trend will continue so you can walk more places!

While I will push for walking, I am not going to go all rabid exerciser on you and push you to go to the next level: biking to work. Many people just aren't up for that. Between having to worry about sweating through your work clothes, to biking in extreme weather, to the danger of cars, there are plenty of reasons to be hesitant to bike. If you are up for it, however, you can cover a lot of ground quickly and will probably have a great time.

At the very least, find a way to integrate walking into your routine. Here are a few ideas - see if any of these strike your fancy:

Errands: Try walking, instead of driving, to run your errands. The store that is a 5 minute drive away is probably not that long of a walk. It may seem like a universe away since you've only ever driven, but put your shoes on and try walking there. You may have a great time when you slow down enough to actually look around at your neighborhood. Even better, carrying groceries or bags home is a workout in itself!

Social walks: Turn a leisurely stroll into a recreational activity. If you have a significant other, hold their hand and walk around romantically. If you have friends, walk and talk. There is something special about conversations on walks: the pressure of having to say something drops away, because even if nobody is speaking, you still have the activity of putting one foot in front of the other to break up the silence. These are even more valuable after meals, and used to be called "constitutionals" because of their health benefits. Walking after a meal not only helps you feel less stuffed, but actually accelerates weight loss. For those of you "show me the science folks," there is a not so creatively titled NIH article called "Walking just after a meal seems to be more effective for weight loss than waiting for one hour to walk after a meal[21]". Start there and keep reading - this kind of study has been done dozens of times with similar results. Those old ladies walking around the block with their goofy visors and fanny packs are definitely onto something.

Get a dog: Dogs take things a step further because they actually get excited to go walking. Some are so jazzed about it that if you even say the w-a-l-k word they'll start jumping up and down in excitement. Dogs need consistent walks to stay healthy. Think about that for a minute. Why would humans not be the same way? Knowing another creature's health is at stake might be a good incentive, unless you're just sadistic. A dog will keep you honest and give you a reason to walk more. Plus, imagine all the friends you'll make with all the other dog-walkers!

Read and walk. Do not do this if you are walking on roads with cars. This is a bad idea unless you are on pedestrian-only paths. However, if there are no cars around, this isn't as hard as it sounds. I've knocked out hundreds of pages over the years while walking, and have yet to have a dangerous incident. Pay attention and you'll probably be fine. For those students out there, studying and walking is also very effective because you have to really focus on thinking about the concepts and not using the written material as a crutch. In college, I found great success by carrying a notecard in my pocket with key points or formulas on it and quizzing myself while walking around campus. This isn't as crazy as it sounds. The best learning happens when you are quizzed, so limiting your materials to those you can read while walking forces you to actually recall things.

Mark here - I can't endorse the read and walk idea. Try it if you like, but be careful!

Walk for creativity. While it has been a common habit of many writers to go on long walks for centuries, in 2014, Stanford psychologists were actually able to quantify this. Their paper, titled "Give Your Ideas Some Legs: The Positive Effect of

Walking on Creative Thinking[22]", found that walking, even if it was indoors on a treadmill, had a positive effect on creativity. There is still speculation on why exactly this is, with some writers noting that walking is similar to meditation because it gets you into a rhythm of steps[23]. Regardless of exactly why, this is another point in defense of walking.

Walking time is not dead time unless you choose to waste it.

Finally, I'll leave you with one last plug on walking. Walking is the oldest, easiest, and cheapest form of travel. Travel doesn't have to mean going to far off places. It can mean taking a different route home, or discovering an interesting house a few blocks away. Travel means discovery, and discovery can happen anywhere. There is a whole world out there, and a lot of it is right in front of you. Go out there and find it! You might just burn a few calories along the way.

Mark here - Henry is 100% correct on the merits of walking. I've averaged 3-5 miles per day since I was a kid. I've had fewer illnesses and fewer aches and pains than most people. Several meniscus and ACL tears prevent me from running, but never slowed me down at all when walking.

CHAPTER 12: LIVE, FAST, AND DIE OLD

◆ ◆ ◆

As weird as this may sound, the best diet I've ever done was also one of the easiest. It was one of the most effective, and one I am sometimes sad I don't do anymore. No, nothing went wrong - at least in the traditional sense. I just don't do it often because it makes me lose weight too fast, and right now, most of my time is spent maintaining weight for lifting.

This diet is called intermittent fasting, and it is amazing. I'm going to try my hardest to not do a deep science review or turn this into a book on fasting, because you'll find hours of content that is more informative than me on the internet and in other publications. My goal is to explain how I did it, why I enjoyed it so much, why I think it worked so well, and what we can learn from it even if we decide not to practice fasting itself.

I did the 16-8 fast, meaning that I would fast 16 hours per 24 hour day and eat 8. The typical recommendation here is simply to skip breakfast and start eating around lunch time, but keep a constant eating window throughout the week. I played around with 12pm to 8pm and 2pm to 10pm eating windows and saw no meaningful difference between them.

Day one of fasting started off on a blissful note when I realized that the extra 30 minutes I needed to grab and eat breakfast was instantly freed up - poof! I used this time for joyous sleep instead. It was strange not eating, but no harm no foul.

By noon (I wasn't eating until 2), I was starving. Like "tackle a random guy walking down the street with a hamburger and eat it in his face" starving. Luckily for me, I didn't have food with or near me and was absorbed in my work. I soldiered on, pausing a few times to question why I was doing this stupid diet, but I stayed strong.

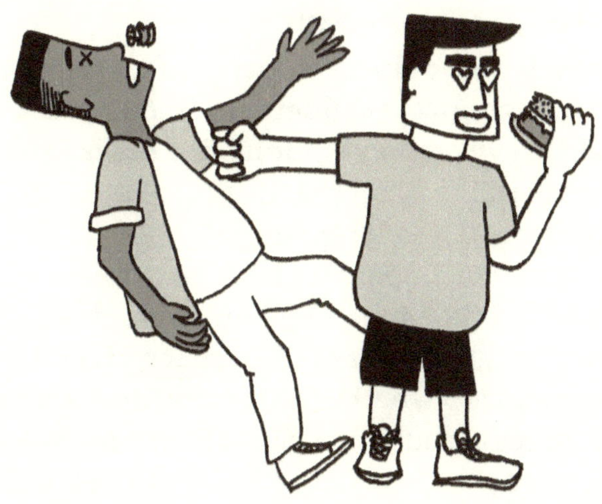

30 minutes later, it was like a switch flipped.

Suddenly the hunger was gone. I felt focused and at ease. For the next few hours, there was no hunger at all. The only sense I can make of it is that my body realized I wasn't giving it any food for fuel and said "fine, I'll turn on the backup generators" and started using good old-fashioned body fat instead. My body protested strongly beforehand, when I was ready to hamburgle, but it quickly realized it wasn't getting a meal any time soon and stopped distracting me with hunger pangs. It was incredibly liberating realizing that my hunger, though it feels like it is a signal that my body is about to fall apart, is really just the body's way of telling me it is unhappy to have to use its energy reserves.

The hunger came back in a few hours, as if my body was saying "ok pal, seriously, feed me." The whole ritual taught me that I wasn't as dependent on food as I seemed.

There is something serene about fasting, and there is a reason many religions practice it as a way to show piety. Part of the serenity comes from allowing your body to focus on something other than eating and digesting for a change. So much of our culture is built around constant eating. If someone finds out you skipped a meal, they often become concerned. Don't let society's expectations dictate your behavior here - you will be absolutely fine if you miss one meal!

There is no way we would have gotten to where we are today as a species if humans in the wilderness 20,000 years ago withered away and died when they couldn't find breakfast. Once you let your body take a break on the digestion, it can dedicate its focus to other things like cell repair.

If you have some time, spend an hour on the internet looking into the health benefits of fasting. You might be amazed with what you find. Though early as of the writing of this book, there are studies looking into whether fasting improves cancer treatment and outcomes because it starves the cancer cells while allowing your body to eat its own body fat instead of food. Even places like Harvard are starting to look into fasting now[24].

Keep in mind that while many researchers swear by it, some sources claim that fasting is no more valuable than traditional calorie restriction diets[25]. Though the formal "science" has yet to reach a conclusion, it was extremely effective for me and gave me one of the most valuable things in the universe: extra time. For some people, it works like a charm, while others are not fans.

Try it, and see if you like it.

The best part of fasting is the sublime carnage that ensues when you you break the fast. Since by the time I got around to eating, I'd missed my entire morning of meals, I was in a big caloric deficit. Sometimes before my first bite I wasn't actually hungry, since my stomach hadn't come back for its second hunger pang, but the second I tasted food, I suddenly became starving. No matter what the food was, it tasted unbelievably good.

I remember breaking my fast with unflavored broccoli and it tasting like a Michelin-star meal. I had a great time breaking my fasts because in addition to everything tasting wonderful, I legitimately had to eat an inhumanly large portion to make sure I got enough daily food in. By compressing my eating window into a smaller time period, I was forced to see just how much food I was eating.

Now, after a few weeks of fasting, things started getting interesting. I went from having the blurry outline of abs to very sharp abs, without any additional changes other than meal timing. It was incredible. To be clear, while this was somewhat magical since I didn't change what I ate, only manipulating the meal timing for these results, I did start with a relatively healthy base of foods that focused on lean meats, veggies, and complex carbs. If you do intermittent fasting entirely with horrendously sugary desserts, the results may not be nearly as good.

No matter where you are starting from, one trick you should try is starting your eating window with the most nutritious, least tasty foods. Hack your body and give your fasted self all the veggies you don't really want to eat first so you'll pack in the nutrients in and fill your stomach. The beauty of fasting is that it compresses your eating window, and means your stomach is only in business for a certain amount of hours per day. Especially if you are eating nutrient-dense, natural foods, there is only so much volume of food you can pack into your stomach in an 8 hour window. Fasting exploits this and gives you a wonderful feeling of extreme fullness since you are trying to pack a full day's food into half the time, so you feel less deprived.

It is worth experimenting with dropping to even shorter than 8 hour eating windows to maximize this effect. Imagine if you had only 45 minutes to get a full day's calories in: you would be brutally efficient and would stick to the good stuff.

Why Snacking is Dumb

Maybe you hate fasting. Maybe it gets you nauseous and ruins your ability to focus. While I think you should stick it out and keep at it for a few more days to see if things get easier, even if you don't, there's an important lesson here:

Less meals mean less calories.

The dieting industry has convinced people that the best way to lose weight is to eat a bunch of tiny meals throughout the day, to graze instead of having a few big meals. I call baloney on the idea that more meals helps you eat less. Major baloney. It makes perfect sense that you'll need more meals if a nutrition company wants you to buy its meal replacement supplements, however.

After doing fasting for a few months and getting wonderfully lean, I realized that I wanted to pack on some weight again to make it easier to get stronger in the gym. I tried to add in more food to my intermittent fasting diet, but found that I was so painfully full during my eating window that I couldn't get down any more calories, and I wasn't willing to cram in junk food to get more calories.

Anecdotally, when I want to gain weight for lifting now, I add more meals. Each meal is less of an event, and doesn't fill me up that much. I am in a constant state of hunger, or at least not total fullness. I find that I can eat dramatically more calories by having more meals, and think less of each individual meal. This is exactly what snacking is: little pieces of food throughout the day that you forget about but add in extra calories that seem inconsequential.

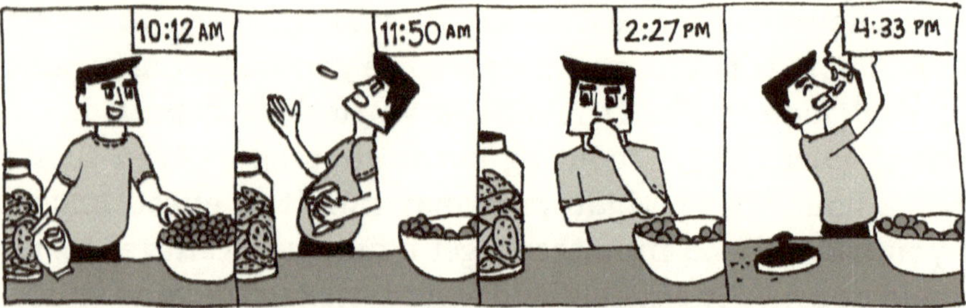

Oops, turns out they aren't, and suddenly you're a bit squishier than you expected without even being any more full.

Even worse is the fact that most snacks are nutritionally not useful on their own. You have the salty and crunchy variety, which are mostly carb and fat-heavy and often calorically dense without being very filling, and then you have the sweet variety, which are usually just a lot of carbs. You may argue that a snack is just a hundred or two hundred calories: what damage can that do? In a day, not much. But add that up over months and years, remembering that a pound of fat is 3,500 calories, and you may be going down a slippery slope.

Remember, we're setting up a diet for the rest of our lives. Everything has to be in the context of sustainability over the next few decades.

That said, there are some snacks that may truly be harmless. Munching on kale or carrots is not likely to do much damage. You can dig up dozens of healthy snacks that don't make a big impact nutritionally and you don't hate eating, but those would still be the small minority of all the snacks out there. They would likely be expensive and either hard to find in stores or have to be home-made. They wouldn't be the easy snacks all around tempting you day in and day out. You could play this game with your healthy snacks, or you could go with the simplest solution and just decide you aren't going to snack at all.

Eat a real meal like an adult that has things like protein and vegetables in it. Snacks are for babies and children that are growing so fast that if they don't eat it will stunt their growth. If you need snacks, you are either not eating enough at your normal meals, or are just babying your body. Stop eating them for a while and see what happens.

One clarification to add: having more meals is not always bad, even for weight loss. I have done plenty of very successful diets where I had 4-6 meals per day. However, doing that requires careful attention to portion sizes. For simplicity purposes, especially if you are new to dieting, you may find more success with fewer total meals, and fasting can be a great low-thought way to do that. As you become more advanced in dieting, you may find that you do better with more meals. Most importantly, don't be dogmatic about it, and don't snack (eat meals without nutritional value).

Mark here - I feel my best when I eat breakfast, lunch, and dinner with little to no snacking. I dispute the notion of "grazing" all day to avoid being hungry. You won't lose weight with a grazing strategy, think about it.

Recently, I've experimented with eating all of my food within 8 hours each day, in my example between 10:30 am and 6:30 pm (I did have coffee with milk before 10:30 and possibly some red wine after 6:30). Given that this data is a sample of 1 and for only a few weeks, but I found I could eat quite a bit more than normal and not gain any weight. Count me a believer in the 8 hour eating window concept. I have no idea if a shorter window would be better. I wouldn't enjoy it.

It is a common stereotype about older people eating early for the early bird special. Until recently, as a Florida resident myself, I joked about that along with everyone else. However, early bird pricing aside, I've found that as I've gotten older, I sleep better when I eat dinner earlier. I don't know the science behind this, but it is true.

CHAPTER 13: THE FAT AND HAPPY SCALE

◆ ◆ ◆

If you've gotten this far in the book, you have tried cutting out sugary drinks, sleeping more, walking more, weighing yourself, and fasting, and still haven't made the progress you want. Or maybe you're just looking for more ideas to have in your back pocket. Either way, things are about to get serious. We're going to dive into the mechanism of how your body changes, and how much it hates change. This will help explain, if you are not making progress, what might be stopping you.

Your body loves where it is. Any change makes it slightly uncomfortable, and drastic changes make it very unhappy. You may have heard the argument before: this is an evolutionary adaptation. If you lose a bunch of weight, your body assumes it is in a famine and times are tough, so whenever it gets the chance, it will gain the weight back as soon as possible. I think of this relationship as what I call the "Fat and Happy Scale" which shows that your body is happiest in equilibrium.

Equilibrium is that point you bounce back to once you stop dieting and go back to your normal eating or life habits. It is the weight you've been fluctuating around for years. Some people may have a changing equilibrium, or have larger fluctuations than others, but there will usually be a weight that your body naturally gravitates to. That is your equilibrium.

Behold, the scale:

Happiness*	1	3	5	4	2
Location	Lean and Unhappy (LU)	Lean and Happy (LH)	Equilibrium (EQ)	Fat and Happy (FH)	Fat and Unhappy (FU)

1 being the least happy, 5 being the most happy

In our chart, notice the edges - at fat and unhappy, your happiness is still higher than lean and unhappy. It isn't fun being so heavy that walking is dangerous on your joints and your body is becoming diabetic and cancerous, but your body prefers that to starvation. Hence, there is a positive skew to the side of gaining weight. Your body would prefer to be at equilibrium, but if that isn't possible, it would be happier gaining weight than losing it.

Thank goodness for this - it is nature's form of insurance and gives us instincts to pack on extra weight in good times so we will last longer in bad times. It has essentially turned our bodies into battery packs, only instead of electricity, we are storing calories.

Now, notice the gray parts of the scale. Your body prefers equilibrium, but it is still relatively happy (or at least lukewarm) with small changes away from it. It still skews towards the fat side, but is ok with being slightly leaner than equilibrium.

The key here is slightly. Your body is like the proverbial frog in boiling water. If you throw a frog in boiling water, just as if you try to rapidly lose or gain a lot of weight, the body will say "this sucks, I'm out" and fight back with extreme cravings or feelings of fullness until your bodyweight jumps back to equilibrium, just like the frog will jump out. However, if you put the frog in room temperature water (equilibrium), and slowly change the temperature, it won't notice the difference until it is too late and it will get cooked.

That is exactly what we are trying to do with our bodies: trick them into changing their equilibrium weight by losing it nice and slowly.

Disclaimer: I have never actually cooked a live frog so don't know if it really works this way. This is just an analogy. I have eaten frogs, however. If cooked right, they can be very tasty. If cooked poorly, they taste like swamp water.

To illustrate how this happens, the chart below simplifies the fat and happy scale, removing the lean and happy and fat and happy pieces. The previous scale was all relative to equilibrium, with the outer edges meaning relatively fat/lean and unhappy compared to where you are now. The scale below is more absolute, with the far left edge representing someone who is absolutely lean and unhappy, meaning the leanest they could be without dying.

Lean and Unhappy									Fat and Unhappy
Too lean									Too fat

For men, this minimum leanness is somewhere south of 6-8% body fat. For women, this is somewhere below 12%. The exact numbers are hard to pin down, with a lot of estimates floating around, and may vary by person, but the key is that this is where you cut into your essential fat stores, where the body becomes so lean that its immune system becomes compromised.

This level of leanness is where professional bodybuilders spend the last few weeks before a competition, and where a lot of their photos are taken: at a level they look inhuman because there is virtually no fat on them.

Being this lean absolutely sucks. Not only is your immune system compromised, but your body's glycogen (energy) stores are depleted, and your hormones can get out of whack. For women, this can result in what is called athletic amenorrhea, or "the term used for when you don't have menstrual periods because you have been exercising very intensely and are very lean[26]". Regardless of gender, being this lean means you are exhausted, cranky, and likely to get sick. Because of that, most bodybuilders don't stay there very long, and quickly add some fat back after their competition. Nobody stays in "contest shape" year-round.

Don't worry. This does not mean you can't be lean enough to consistently have abs and look great while still being healthy! Being a few percentage body fat points above this unhealthy level is something you can maintain. This is represented by the box just to the right of the orange "Lean and Unhappy" box.

On the other end of the spectrum, in the "Fat and Unhappy" box, you have someone who is as fat as they can be without dying. This is difficult to put an exact number on, but represents the point where someone's health and mobility is impaired because of their weight and body fat. They are carrying around so many pounds that even walking is exhausting. Their joints ache under the load of their weight. Their heart has to pump a lot more blood than the heart of a smaller person. Their body has so much body fat that it has trouble maintaining blood sugar levels, and is likely developing, or already has, Type II Diabetes. At this weight, someone is at very high risk for a heart attack and their weight is hindering their everyday life.

Remember, this is just a representation of an extreme, not an actual scientific scale. This point will be a different weight for everyone, and in truth, it doesn't matter where exactly this limit is. What matters is that it exists, and that there is a lot of room between the limits to play around in.

A limit of being too lean exists as well, with the area past these limits representing health problems. Where these points are exactly matter less than the idea that there are definite boundaries to a healthy weight or body composition.

Now that we've established that there is a maximum level of leanness and a maximum level of fatness that someone can be and still be healthy, we have the huge area between them to play around in.

It is beyond the scope of this book to tell you how lean someone should be for optimum health, and a lot of opinions are out there. I am assuming everyone has a goal state in mind. Earlier, we talked about looking like the cover model on a fitness magazine. Maybe that is where you want to be. Maybe you just want to be a little thinner. Regardless of what you goal is, the concept to achieve it will be the same: you need to slowly move your equilibrium. In this case, I will assume someone is moving it to the left, to a leaner equilibrium, but the same concept is similar for someone trying to gain weight and move to the right (yes, those people exist - talk to most male contact sport athletes!).

The chart below shows a time series of what you might think the your weight loss trajectory would be: every time period (time passes as you move down the chart) you move your equilibrium slightly leaner.

LU									EQ		FU
LU								EQ			FU
LU							EQ				FU
LU						EQ					FU
LU					EQ						FU
LU				EQ							FU
LU			EQ								FU
LU		EQ									FU
Too lean											Too fat

You would do this by slowly pushing your body to the lean and happy zone, just slightly dropping your calories to make an incremental drop in weight. A 15% drop in calories is the number often thrown around as the maximum you should decrease at once, and serves as a good guidepost. For some people, they'll see results with more like a 10% decrease, while others can operate with more like a 20% decrease.

If this were how the world works, we'd end the book here and everyone would leave happy. However, a real progression often looks jagged and winding, more like the following chart:

LU							EQ		FU
LU						EQ			FU
LU						EQ			FU
LU					EQ				FU
LU				EQ					FU
LU					EQ				FU
LU				EQ					FU
LU			EQ						FU
LU		EQ							FU
LU	EQ								FU
LU	EQ								FU
Too lean									Too fat

There are ups and downs. Sometimes you make great progress, and sometimes your body just decides "nope, I want to go back to the way it was." Your body is less like a normal frog and more like a frog that sometimes comes back to life on your dinner plate and has to be thrown back into the pot and boiled. It can be very tenacious. All you can do is keep playing the long game and fighting the good fight.

For better or for worse, the more time your body spends in one equilibrium ("set point"), the more comfortable it gets there, and the more it cements that weight as one it will come back to without conscious effort. This can be a double-edged sword. If you are at the weight you want to be, it is a blessing: the longer you stay at that weight, the easier that weight is to maintain. If you are far from your ideal weight, it is a curse, because the longer you stay where you are, the harder it is to move to where you want to be. It is as if the gravitational pull grows stronger with every day you stay where you are.

Your first reaction to hearing about the set point may be: "I need to lose weight as fast as possible!". This is logical and how most people approach dieting. But there is a better way: not focusing on losing weight as fast as possible, but focusing on losing it as persistently as possible. It a persistent effort to move to the left on the scale, and even when things backslide, getting back in the saddle and continuing to move the needle.

To be clear, this is an oversimplification. We know you won't make progress every day or every month, and that is ok. Don't beat yourself up. You need to embrace that and plan to stall sometimes. Let your body feel a new set point and reset to a lower body weight. Resetting is a many-week process, and will vary based on your body's circumstances. Try four-week resets, where you stay at a lower weight for a month before losing weight again. This would make your progression look like the below chart (assuming each box is a month):

LU							EQ		FU
LU						EQ			FU
LU						EQ			FU
LU					EQ				FU
LU					EQ				FU
LU				EQ					FU
LU				EQ					FU
LU			EQ						FU
LU			EQ						FU
LU		EQ							FU

If you feel like four-week resets are not long enough, try six or eight weeks. Even if you are just maintaining, that is progress because you are maintaining at a lower set point. Keep boiling that frog.

Mark here - I like Henry's concept of equilibrium but want to interject a counter-idea. I believe that your weight is rarely in equilibrium. Instead you are always either gaining or losing. I've noticed that when you been losing weight you can overeat and still lose weight for a day or so before you start gaining. Conversely, when you've been gaining, it takes several days of under eating before you start to lose weight. The trend can be your friend or your enemy.

Henry here - my dad's counter-idea is an important nuance to my equilibrium idea. Think of equilibrium as a long term, slow-moving average, with a lot of noisy fluctuations around it in the short term. What this means for you is to keep calm and carry on for a few days, even if you change your behavior and nothing seems to change immediately. The momentum will shift over time. If you forget all the specifics of the charts, remember that long term consistency is what matters most.

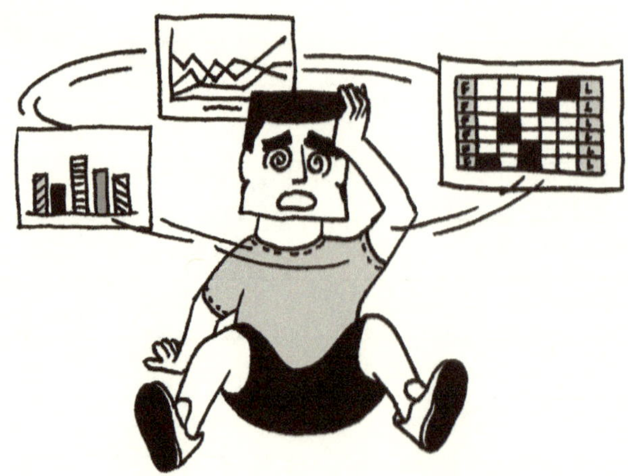

CHAPTER 14: WHAT TO EAT

◆ ◆ ◆

Congratulations, you made it. You've graduated past lifestyle changes into dietary changes. This chapter will feel more like most dieting books, because we are going to talk about specific foods.

You could spend the rest of your life reading detailed diet books on what exactly you should be eating. Organic for some fruits, but not for others. Herbal tea at a certain time of day. This veggie, but only if blended or sautéed, not grilled. Grass fed beef. Wild salmon, but not mackerel. Free range eggs. Are you overwhelmed yet? Let's take a few steps back.

All of these considerations are relevant, and there is plenty of science behind them. However, worrying about them as obsessively as most people do, without getting the basics right, is like getting your shoes polished but forgetting to put on your pants and shirt. It is great, but just a small little detail that matters far less than the rest of the outfit.

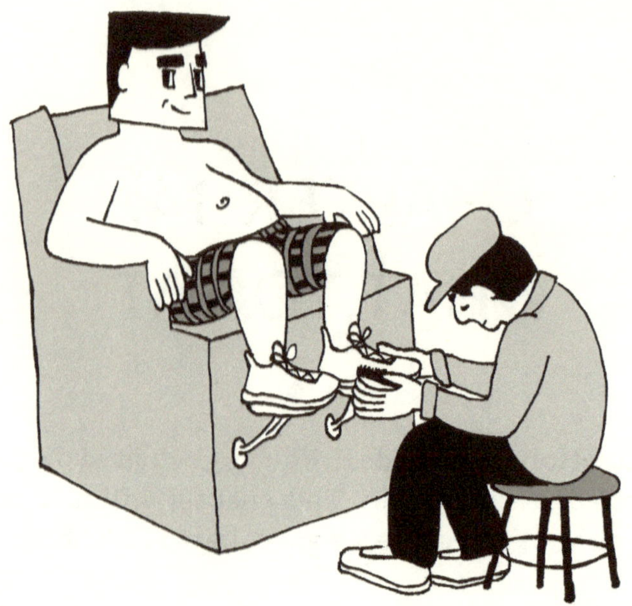

A company called Renaissance Periodization has created a very helpful visual to show what I think really matters when dieting:

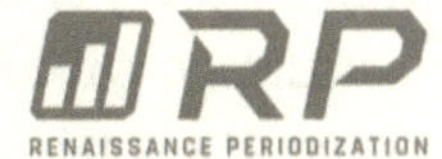

Fig. 1

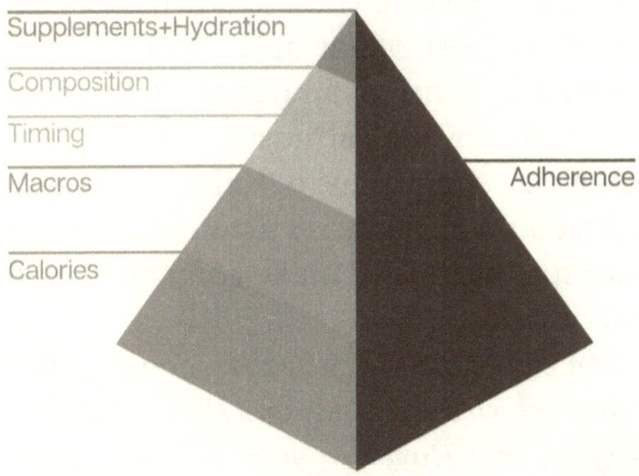

Source: The Renaissance Diet 2.0 by Dr. Mike Israetel, Dr. Melissa Davis, Dr. Jenn Case, and Dr. James Hoffman. Image reproduced with permission. Renaissance Periodization creates books, coaching templates, diet templates, and other resources to help people achieve their physique goals. I do not receive any compensation from them, but have had success using their products, and learned a lot from their content. They are very smart and can take you deep into the weeds of precise science and nutrient counts for you, if you are looking for that.

If you look at this chart, all the pieces about whether you should be eating organic or not, or how you cook your veggies, fit under "food composition", which represents a mere FIVE PERCENT of the total picture.

Far more important than those things are calorie balance and macronutrients ("macros": the amounts of protein, fat, carbohydrates you eat). If you can get your calorie balance and macros right, you're 80% of the way there. For most people, who are just looking to get in better shape, not trying to be ready for a bodybuilding competition, that 80% will get the job done.

The takeaway is that you should spend less time worrying about the nuances and focus on getting the big picture correct.

However, there is one wrinkle to the chart. The 5% for food

composition is slightly more important than it seems because it has a big influence on the other factors. Food composition, or whether you are eating a cup of rice to get 200 calories, or whether you are ingesting these calories through a sugary drink, can impact the other variables. Even though both of those foods have very similar amounts of calories and even macronutrients (they are both almost entirely carbohydrates), the rice will keep you slightly more full than the sugary drink. A few hours later, you'll be hungrier if you had the sugary drink, making it harder to continue to make good choices about macronutrients and calories.

Mark here - You could lose weight eating donuts, it's true. If you ate 3 donuts at 400 calories every day and NOTHING else, you would lose weight pretty quickly. However, you would feel starvation, you would feel terrible, and long term, you would be ill. It won't work, but feel free to experiment. I don't mean to pick on the purveyors of donuts, but I think you will agree that eating a donut doesn't keep you feeling full for very long. A donut is a sugary carb and sugary carbs don't provide satiety. You need some combination of protein and carbs to provide an acceptable level of satiety.

To succeed at consuming few enough calories to lose weight, you have to eat foods that provide a lot of satiety. Your food choices have to satisfy you and fend off hunger pains, at least to a degree. You will still be hungry, but think of hunger as your friend. Hunger is telling you that your body is burning its stored fat.

Henry here - This is one thing to be cognizant of if you are trying the popular If It Fits In Your Macros ("IIFYM") diet, which allows you to eat any kind of food you want as long as you get the right number of calories and amounts of protein, fats, and carbs. A lot of people lIIFYM because it allows them to eat desserts and all the treats they love, which is great, if they can stick to it.

However, things get tricky with IIFYM for two reasons.

First, it is really hard to actually get healthy macros through unhealthy food. You will likely have to do a feast or famine approach, eating only really tasty things (cookies) and really unexciting things (chicken breast and spinach).

Second, once you start having these unhealthy foods, it is hard for your body to not crave more, and they usually are simply not as satiating as healthier foods. As mentioned earlier in the book, many dietitians talk about these cravings coming from sugar messing up your gut bacteria[27], making you crave more of it. I haven't done much gut bacteria study, but at the highest level, it makes sense: you'll want to eat things that you're used to eating.

If you can do IIFYM and not get derailed by these obstacles, by all means, have your cake and eat it too. However, a lot of people will struggle to do that, and find that over time, actually eating healthier more consistently is a more sustainable way to get where they want to be.

So let's go back to the chart above. Adherence is not a part of the pyramid itself, because it truly is the entire thing. If you aren't adhering to the diet, the nuances don't matter. This has to come first, and ties back to the Diet Sustainability Matrix. You need to build a system you enjoy enough to do for the rest of your life.

Do you really want to live your life one 8-week fad diet at a time? Do you want to remember years by whether you were doing a juice cleanse or going no-carb? I didn't think so. Let's keep it simple and make it less excruciating than most diets. My father and I have slightly different approaches to what exactly you can and can't eat. Let's look at his first.

Mark here - Contrary to popular advice, while you are aggressively trying to lose weight, I suggest you eat a fairly narrow range of foods. Choose foods that you like and that don't make you feel bad. I suggest a list for each meal that you rotate.

Foods to eat: *I like foods that fill me up, satisfy cravings, and I like to use a lot of seasoning to offset lower portions.*
Meat - 4 oz or smaller portion sizes
Eggs - Not more than 1 per day
Whole wheat bread - 1 slice per day
Whole wheat crackers - small quantities

Vegetables - any kind
Beans - any kind, but not refried!
Potatoes, rice, other grains - stick to portion size
Red wine - You must measure this as well! A serving is 5 ounces.
Coffee

Foods to never eat! *(Ok, eat rarely). No science here, just my own experience.*
French fries
Potato chips / pretzels
Pizza
Beer
Rum
Soda
Nuts - too many calories, unless you eat the recommended portion size - nobody does!
Artificial sweeteners of every kind.
Cakes, cookies, packaged desserts of any kind.
Fruit- I know it sounds weird to include fruit on the list of foods to avoid or eat sparingly. Eating fruit is much better than eating any kind of processed snack, but fruits still have quite a few calories, eating fruit isn't calorie free and the calories count against your daily totals.
Packaged and processed food in general.

Henry here again - I generally agree with my Dad's thinking on good or bad foods. I think his portion sizes are too small for everyone, even though they work for him, but the gist is spot on. I also agree that a narrow range of food can be helpful, simply because it makes it easier for you to have consistency in what you eat, making it easier to isolate your variables of and tweak them to achieve the results you want. My three exceptions to my dad's recommended food and fruit, nuts, and the idea of banning foods in general:

Fruit: I agree that it has calories that you should keep in mind, but as mentioned in the "Start with Soda" chapter, I personally think fruit is a good substitute for truly dangerous desserts because it hits your sweet tooth while also providing fiber and a lot less calories.

Nuts: I agree that they have a lot of calories, but if used in responsible portion sizes, they can add important fat, satiety, and fiber to a meal.

Banning foods in general: I shy from an explicit ban, not because I think you should eat all the terrible things that we all agree should be banned, but because I worry that permanently banning stuff will make your diet psychologically harder to maintain over a lifetime. If you are strong enough to actually ban things, go for it. But if you can't bear the thought of never eating a cookie again, skip the ban.

So, to be clear, from my perspective, there are no foods you can't eat, with the exception of sugary drinks (see the "Start with Sugary Drinks" chapter). You don't even have to get a certain macro breakdown.

We're going to keep things simple, outlining a spectrum from good to bad food combinations. If you move in the correct direction, from right to left, on that food scale, your macros will improve on their own simply because you are eating healthier items.

That may take care of your weight loss on its own, without the need for you weigh every grain of rice. If after that, you decide that you are super fit and looking to do a bodybuilding competition, or just love measuring things, it may be time to get more precise with your food measurements. But if you prefer to just live your life and not spend a lot of time thinking about food, you can be simply aware of the spectrum and things will sort themselves out on their own. Behold, the food spectrum:

1	2	3	4	5	6	7	8	9
Lean meat, veggies	Lean meat, veggies, complex carbs	Lean meat, veggies, complex carbs, nuts	Fatty meat, veggies, complex carbs	Fatty meat, complex carbs	Fried meats	(Fried) savory nonmeats	Desserts	Sugary drinks
Healthiest								Unhealthiest

Before we get into what to do with what is on the scale, a few definitions are below. Along with each definition, I have provided a table with calories and macronutrients for 100 grams of five common foods within each category. This should help give a sense of caloric density and what macronutrients each category provides. To be clear, I am providing these tables to give you a general understanding of the qualities of a type of foods, not to point you to specific ones within each table. Think of these tables as for illustrative purposes of the food category in general rather than being prescriptive. They are all sourced from standard online nutrition fact data[28] and are meant to be directional guideposts rather than precise recommendations.

Lean meat: Lean meat means any cut of meat with less than 10 grams of fat per 3 ounce serving[29]. This means things like chicken breast, ground meat that is 90% or more lean, pork loin, beef sirloin, beef filet, shrimp, scallops, grouper, halibut, tilapia. This is not an exhaustive list, but the idea is meat without much fat on it. Lean meat is great because it has a lot of protein per ounce without much fat, meaning it is very filling and nourishing without being very high in calories.

The table below gives you an idea of calories and macronutrient content for 100 grams of cooked amounts of a few common types of lean meats. Lean meats, as you can see, are primarily protein with varying amounts of fat.

Item	Calories	Protein	Carbs	Fats
Pork Loin	116	21.6	0.3	3.2
Halibut	140	26.7	0	2.9
Chicken Breast	165	31	0	3.6
Beef Sirloin	193	26.3	0	9.7
90% Ground Beef	230	28.5	0	12

Vegetables: We all know what vegetables ("veggies") are, but they are not all created equal. Things like potatoes and corn do not count - they are considered complex carbs. Spend a few minutes on Google to see which veggies are more nutritious, but the key here is finding some that you like and finding ways to cook them. Veggies have three main purposes. First, they fill you up with a lot of volume but a minimum of calories. Second, they have lots of vitamins that keep your immune system humming along. This is really important - getting sick sucks, and veggies protect you from that. Third, they have fiber for...you should Google "fiber" if you don't know what it is good for.

The table below gives you an idea of calories and macronutrient content for 100 grams of cooked amounts of common veggies. As you can see, veggies are relatively low calories, low fat, with a small amount of carbs (a lot of that is coming from fiber), making them perfect to fill you up without adding a lot of calories.

Item	Calories	Protein	Carbs	Fats
Spinach	23	3	3.7	0.3
Mushroom	26	3.6	4	0.3
Broccoli	28	3.1	5.3	0.1
Bell Pepper	28	0.9	6.7	0.2
Carrots	35	0.8	8.2	0.2

Complex Carbs: For our purposes, complex carbohydrates represent all carb-heavy sources that you have to chew and don't have added sugar. This means fruits, beans, rice, pasta, bread, potatoes, and all other grains, and does not include fruit juice (see "Sugary Drinks" for more on fruit juice). I am defining this far looser than most people, who often consider complex carbohydrates to only be things like beans, brown rice, sweet potatoes, quinoa, and all those mysterious "ancient grains" that the health food stores continue to charge impressively high prices for.

To be clear, not all carbohydrates are the same, and they all have different glycemic indices (Google that if you want to go a layer deeper), but they all play the same general role: carbs provide energy to your body, and fill you up, as they are not that calorically dense. If you had to order them in terms of what is best to eat, beans and lentils take the crown for being highest in fiber and protein, with rice, pasta, and fruit in the middle, and bread on the lower end of the spectrum. However, the differences are not huge, so do not agonize over them.

The table below gives you an idea of calories and macronutrient content for 100 grams of cooked amounts of common complex carbs (except the fruits, which are raw). As you can see, unsurprisingly, complex carbs are all primarily carbohydrates, though some pack more calories per 100 grams than others.

Item	Calories	Protein	Carbs	Fats
Apples	52	0.3	13.8	0.2
Potatoes	97	2.6	21.4	0.1
Lentils	101	8.8	21.2	0.5
White Rice	130	2.7	28.2	0.3
Wheat Bread*	266	10.9	47.5	3.6

*100 grams of wheat bread represents 4 slices, so if you halve that to 2 slices, bread is a lot like the other grain-based complex carbs.

Side Note on Low-Carb Diets

Carbs have gotten a very bad reputation recently, with everyone swearing by low-carb (often called "ketogenic" or "keto") diets.

The idea behind a ketogenic diet is that you drop your carb consumption to a very low level (usually around 30 grams per day), forcing your body to go into what is called ketosis, where your body stops converting carbs to energy and starts converting fat to energy, namely, your body fat.

Sounds great, doesn't it?

Here's the catch. It takes you a few days to fully get into ketosis, and getting there can hurt. Before you can get there, your body has to burn your carb, or glycogen, stores. When they are finally depleted, you will experience something called "hitting a wall", "Atkins flu", or "keto flu," which is when your body reaches total exhaustion and has no more energy available. This is accompanied by multiple days of delightful symptoms like nausea, headache, low-energy, and irritability. Once your body decides to fully transition from its glycogen stores to your body fat for energy, you'll start to feel better.

During this painful carb-depletion process, you will drop weight rapidly. This is because glycogen is very heavy and is comprised of mostly water[30]. When you eat carbs, you will gain weight quickly, but most of it is truly water weight rather than actual body fat. Therefore, many low carb dieters will see huge initial 5-10 pound weight drops in the first few days and declare immediate success. That is the mirage of water-weight.

Additionally, once you get in ketosis, you need to continue eating low-carb to stay in it, or the whole painful process will start all over again. Therefore, you will be forever doomed to be that annoying friend trying to figure out if the salad dressing has any carbs in it.

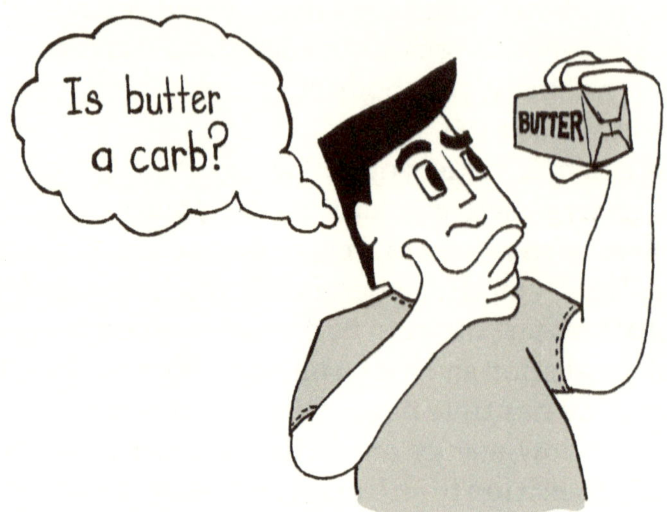

Not only is ketosis painful to get into and socially difficult to maintain, it also doesn't necessarily guarantee success. Once you transition off of carbs to fats for your energy source, you will change your eating to only protein and fats. This means a lot of bacon and fatty meat.

In a way, this can be great, because the fat and protein will keep you very satiated.

However, fat has over double the amount of calories per gram (9 calories per gram of fat compared to around 4 calories per gram of protein or carbohydrate), making it exponentially easier to accidentally scarf down 1,000 calories effortlessly eating fatty foods than leaner ones. Yes, the fat will usually keep you full and away from bingeing too much, but you can still do a lot more caloric damage than you might realize with fatty meats, cheeses, and bacon. For our purposes of keeping things simple and mindless, keto gets a thumbs down because you have to pay a lot of attention to make sure you are not accidentally eating an extra 1,000 calories from fatty meats.

I know this may disappoint some of you. It disappointed me too after I did a keto diet for several months. At the end of it, sure, I had made progress, but no better progress than I had made on far more normal and easier diets. The miraculous promise of more muscle mass that some people claim keto provides never happened to me. While I did lose weight initially, I quickly found a weight equilibrium since I was having so many calories from bacon and sausage. The weight loss wasn't effortless after the initial drop.

Most importantly, I had an incredibly painful time in every single social situation because I could only eat a fraction of the food served with any given meal. This made keto not worth it for me.

Despite all of this, keto diets are still all the rage. What gives? While they do have their downsides, I believe they can be helpful for some people, especially those that are significantly overweight or eat too much sugar. Low carb diets, to their credit, do remove some of the most fattening carb-heavy foods like sugar, pizza, and french fries, which can make a big improvement in someone's dieting progress. This can make them very effective for people who eat a lot of food from the right side of our food spectrum.

However, in my opinion, low carb diets throw out the baby with the bath water, because not all carbs are bad, and avoiding them altogether makes your diet much more difficult to maintain.

Keto will usually help you lose weight if you are significantly overweight. It has helped people conquer obesity. However, even if you do keto, you still have to make sure that you are not overdoing your calories and fats. Cutting carbs can make that easier to do if you are eating huge amounts of junk food and sugar, but just because you are not eating carbs does not mean the other variables don't matter. For this reason, I suggest most people avoid keto and use a more sustainable approach of eating healthier carbs and being mindful of portions.

Fatty Meat: For our simplified purposes, fatty meat will include the usual suspects like fatty ground beef, chuck roast, and chicken thighs, but will also include eggs, fatty fish (trout, salmon, etc.), and organ meats. There is a big range within fatty meats, and if you are interested, you can spend a very long time researching it all online. The bottom line is to beware of just how fatty the meat you're about to eat is, and how processed.

Things like sausage and bologna usually are more fat that protein, and some brands can be packed with chemicals and salt. Check the nutrition facts on things before you get them just to know if you're actually getting any protein or if it is just fat with some protein on top. Sorry bacon, I'm looking at you - you're a side meat, not a main meat.

The three things you might not have expected within fatty meats:

Fatty fish is awesome for you. It is expensive and sometimes smelly to cook at home, so likely won't be a staple in your diet, but is loaded with Omega 3 fatty acids that are good for your heart. While fish oil tablets might be a decent starting point, nutritionists note that they are not as effective as eating actual fish[31]. Just be aware of mercury levels - they can be dangerously high in predatory fish like swordfish[32].

Organ meats, if you can stand the taste, are also loaded with nutrients that are supposedly mind-blowingly healthy[33]. They are also cheap. Interestingly, in other countries and in past centuries, organ meats were often the most coveted pieces of meat, with the steaks being fed to the dogs while the royalty ate the organs. Marketing and social norms have convinced us that they are gross, but nutritionally, we are missing out.

Eggs, despite being boo-hoo'd for decades because of their cholesterol, are now back on the good list. Doctors have recently come around to saying that an average of an egg a day is not harmful and may actually be healthy[34]. Do a Google search for "are eggs healthy" and you'll be happy to read about all the fun nutrients they have in them. More importantly, they are cheap, easy to get, filling and tasty. I concede that their protein to fat ratio isn't ideal, and will often supplement with added egg whites, a more protein-rich meat, or milk to get enough protein in a meal, but eggs are a powerful tool to have in your toolkit. The table below gives you an idea of calories and macronutrient content for 100 grams of cooked amounts of common fatty meats. As you can see, while they all pack a solid protein punch, it often comes with a lot of fat.

Item	Calories	Protein	Carbs	Fats
Eggs	196	13.6	0.9	15.3
Salmon	206	22.1	0	12.3
70/30 Ground Beef	270	25.6	0	17.9
Italian Sausage	344	19.1	4.3	27.3
Bacon	533	38.3	1.5	40.3

Nuts: This refers to nuts that are not coated with sugar or chocolate. Nuts have a wide range of tastes and prices: you can pay $4 per pound of peanuts, or $16 per pound of almonds. Pick your poison. Nuts are great because they are infinitely portable without refrigeration, have lots of healthy fats, and are full of fiber. They are a great way to add in some extra calories and fat to a meal, or to eat on the go. More importantly, they allow you flexibility in your diet in a way that fatty meats don't.

What do I mean by flexibility? Let's say at 2pm you get ambushed by an office birthday party, and someone insists you eat a slice of cake, giving you a lot more fat and carbs that you were expecting. With nuts planned into your next meal, you can just take the nuts and carbs out since you already got a bunch of fat and carbs from the cake, but you'll still get the protein from the lean meat. Fatty meats do not allow the flexibility of breaking apart the fat and protein, allow this flexibility, since the fat and protein go together. We are also including avocado within the nuts category, as it is also full of healthy fat and fiber. There are two caveats to nuts.

First, they do have some protein, and food companies love touting that things like peanut butter are a good source of protein. However, per calorie, nuts are a terrible protein source compared to lean meats. For example, a serving of peanut butter - 2 tablespoons - has 200 calories, and 8 grams of protein, or 0.04 grams of protein per calorie. A serving of baked chicken breast, 4 ounces, has 187 calories and 35 grams of protein, or 0.19 grams of protein per calorie. That means that lean meat has approximately five times the amount of protein per calorie.

Unless you are trying to gain weight very fast, nuts as a protein source are not a good idea, bringing us to our second caveat: nuts are very calorically dense. They are often used by hikers as a trail food because they pack so many calories per pound. It is dangerously easy to accidentally eat 2,000 calories of nuts in one sitting, especially if you get the tasty salted ones. Be very careful with them, and be mindful of your nut portions. I usually stick to 1-3 tablespoons of nuts at a time and measure them carefully. Do not just eat them out of the can without measuring - you will overeat. Nuts may have healthy fats, but overdoing them will just make you overweight and full of healthy fats.

I've found that one of the best uses of nuts is putting them in with your vegetables. If you have salted peanuts with your broccoli, you can almost forget that you're eating broccoli sometimes because of the nice taste and crunch. Make sure you measure how much you are putting in, but don't be afraid to mix nuts with veggies to make the veggies taste better.

You'll notice that we don't include oils here. Sometimes you're going to need oils to complete a recipe, but when given the choice, nuts are a better fat source than oils simply because oils include just the fatty part without the actual fiber. Oils aren't that bad, but they are simply concentrated calories - no chewing required, so nuts are better.

The table below gives you an idea of calories and macronutrient content for 100 grams of raw amounts of common nuts (including avocado). As mentioned, these have high fat content with relatively low protein and carbs. While this is not captured in the table, they also have a solid amount of fiber. Notice that avocado is significantly lower in calories - that is because it has a lot of water in it, which adds volume but not calories. Regardless, avocado is still a high-fat calorie source.

Item	Calories	Protein	Carbs	Fats
Avocado	160	2	8.5	14.7
Cashews	553	18.2	32.7	43.8
Pistachios	557	20.6	28	44.4
Peanuts	567	25.8	16.1	49.2
Almonds	575	21.2	21.7	49.4

Fried Meats: Adding a layer of frying to a meat makes it very tasty, but that comes with both carbohydrates (from the breading on the fry), and fats (from the oil it is fried in). Fried meats can be dangerous because they pack a lot more calories than their non-fried cousins.

To give you an idea, if you are looking to get 35 grams of protein, you can get it from about 112 grams of baked chicken breast, which provides 185 calories, or you can get it from about 140 grams of fried chicken breast, which provides 364 calories. That means frying pretty much doubles the calories.

However, even though frying adds calories, you're still frying a meat, so you still have the protein and sometimes fat of the underlying meat. While not ideal, fried meats will be at least more filling than non-meats and desserts. The table below gives you an idea of calories and macronutrient content for 100 grams of cooked amounts of common fried meats. As you can see, while they do still have protein, it comes with fat and additional carbs, adding a lot more calories.

Item	Calories	Protein	Carbs	Fats
Fried Catfish	229	18.1	8	13.3
Fried Chicken Breast	260	24.8	9	13.2
Fried Chicken Drumstick	268	21.9	8.3	15.7
Fried Chicken Thigh	298	21.8	9.4	18.6

(Fried) savory non-meats: In layman's terms: snacks! French fries, chips, pizza, popcorn, pretzels and anything similar. These items are almost always a tasty way to get fat and carbs in your system, usually with minimal protein. These are slightly better than desserts because they usually don't have sugar in them, but they aren't really doing your body any good. Know that when you are eating these, you're doing it purely for your own enjoyment, and not for any health or fitness benefit.

The table below gives you an idea of calories and macronutrient content for 100 grams of cooked amounts of common (fried) savory non-meats. As you can see, these are primarily carbs and fats, with small amounts of protein.

Item	Calories	Protein	Carbs	Fats
Pizza	264	11.9	32.6	9.5
French Fries	319	3.8	37.5	17.1
Pretzels	381	9.1	79.2	3.5
Popcorn	527	8.7	55.7	30
Potato Chips	547	6.6	49.7	37.5

Desserts: Donuts, cakes, pies, cookies, candy, chocolate, et cetera. These are almost entirely fat and carbs with minimal protein. They also have sugar in them, which will make you hungrier. The only bright side is that at least they are solid food, meaning that you are doing some form of chewing rather than purely drinking your calories, so while you can do a lot of damage quickly, you are at least watching the food go into your mouth and spooning it yourself, which may slow you down. This is also good because solid food will take your body a little bit longer to digest, and fill you up a little bit more than a purely liquid dessert would.

The table below gives you an idea of calories and macronutrient content for 100 grams of common desserts. As noted, these are almost entirely fat and carbs.

Item	Calories	Protein	Carbs	Fats
Vanilla Ice Cream	207	3.5	23.6	11
Jellybeans	375	9	83.5	0.1
Glazed Donut	399	6.2	50.6	19.1
Chocolate Bar	471	5.8	55.1	29.3
Chocolate Chip Cookie	488	5.7	58.2	28.4

Sugary Drinks: Soda, milkshakes, most juices, punch, and the like. These are the baddest of the bad. If you are trying to add thick layers of body fat as fast as possible, you're in the right place! Sugary drinks are like adding kerosene to a fire, with that fire being your hunger. They digest very quickly and you can down incredible amounts of calories without noticing, no chewing needed. Combine that with the addictive effects of sugar, and sugary drinks are the granddaddy of poor diet choices. Hence, my strong recommendation is to avoid sugary drinks altogether.

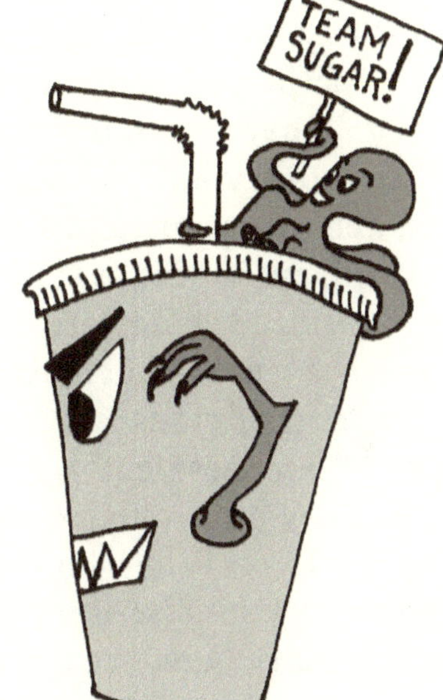

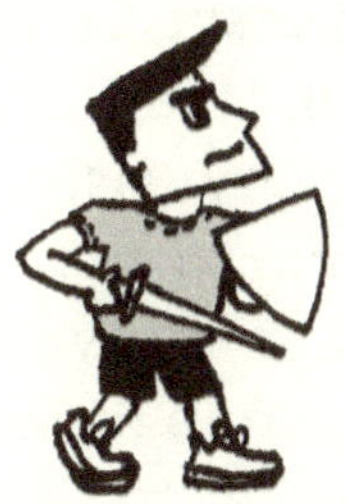

The table below gives you an idea of calories and macronutrient content for 100 grams of common sugary drinks. These are mostly pure carbs, though versions with dairy have fat and a tiny bit of protein as well.

Don't be deceived by the low calorie counts in this table - these are because these are based on 100 gram servings, and liquid is heavy, making them seem less caloric. A 100 gram serving is less than a half cup of these drinks, so you will end up having far more than 100 grams of them without feeling much more full.

Item	Calories	Protein	Carbs	Fats
Soda (Cola)	37	0.1	9.6	0
Orange Juice	44	0.8	10.1	0.3
Apple Juice	46	0.1	11.3	0.1
Fruit Punch	46	0.1	11.7	0
Vanilla Milkshake	155	2.9	20.3	7.5

Forgotten Foods!

In the 9 point spectrum, some things are not listed. The spectrum should capture most things, but some strange or hybrid foods may not fit neatly into these simple categories. Maybe you're perplexed and wondering how to classify some food item you love to eat. If something is missed, do some research and see what your food is closest to as far as calories, ingredients, and macronutrient breakdown with what we've already outlined, and slot it in there. If you're really worried about it, just consider it a dessert, eat it sparingly, and see if eating it causes changes to your body composition.

The most obvious category that is ignored by the spectrum is dairy. Milk, cheese, cottage cheese and yogurt aren't mentioned at all. They are a complicated hybrid that can vary based on whether you get the whole or reduced fat versions, so you will need to use your discretion and make it a choose-your-own-adventure story here. I've left dairy out of the spectrum because if you are trying to keep things simple, dairy is going to throw a wrench in your perfectly functioning simple machine. However, since so many people love it so much, a few points to note as you go on your dairy quest:

Milk can be great. It has calcium, which everyone loves. It has protein, carbs, and fat as well. If you are in a pinch, it can be a great source of sustenance. However, it does have a decent amount of sugar in it, so beware. The protein and fact that the sugar is not artificially added mean milk isn't quite a true "sugary drink", but it isn't perfect either. As such, you probably don't hear about a lot of milk-focused weight-loss diets.

In fact, in weightlifting communities, the GOMAD (gallon of milk a day) diet, which has you downing a jug of whole milk every day, is sometimes recommended to lifters who struggle to gain weight. Spend some time researching results, however, and you'll see that GOMAD isn't exactly the key to abs.

If you love milk and can't live without it, the first solution is to just pay attention to its macronutrients and have a little bit less of other parts of your meal. I personally have some milk every day with my eggs to add in some protein, since eggs don't have that much on their own. I have a little less rice to account for the carbs in the milk, and voila! No harm done.

The second solution is finding ultra-filtered or fortified milks. I actually still am almost skeptical that this stuff is real because it seems too good to be true. There is one popular brand of fortified milk with twice the protein and half the sugar of normal milk. It is done with some protein/sugar separation process (I picture a big centrifuge) that results in it being normal milk just with more good stuff (protein) and less bad stuff (sugar). Amazingly, to me and my parents, who are picky, it doesn't taste noticeably different from normal milk. It also claims to have no lactose, so can be a solution if you are lactose-free. It costs more than regular milk, but seems pretty worth it.

Cheese is one of my favorite foods in the world. It has no carbs, some protein, and a lot of calories and delicious flavor. In the past I have incorporated it into my meals, but generally only when trying to gain weight. I consider it "the lazy man's flavoring" because you can put it on almost anything to improve the taste. I won't say to never have cheese, but be aware of cheese's power and caloric density.

Cheese isn't incredibly unhealthy, and you probably wouldn't do much damage by having it on lean meat, but be conscious of the calories in it. Nuts are superior to cheese as a fat source because they have fiber that will fill you up a bit more and help you have better digestion. Your best use of cheese is likely to enjoy it on occasion but know it isn't really a fit for your everyday meals, but this isn't dogma! If you find a way to eat lots of cheese achieve the results you want, go wild. Remember, the food police aren't real!

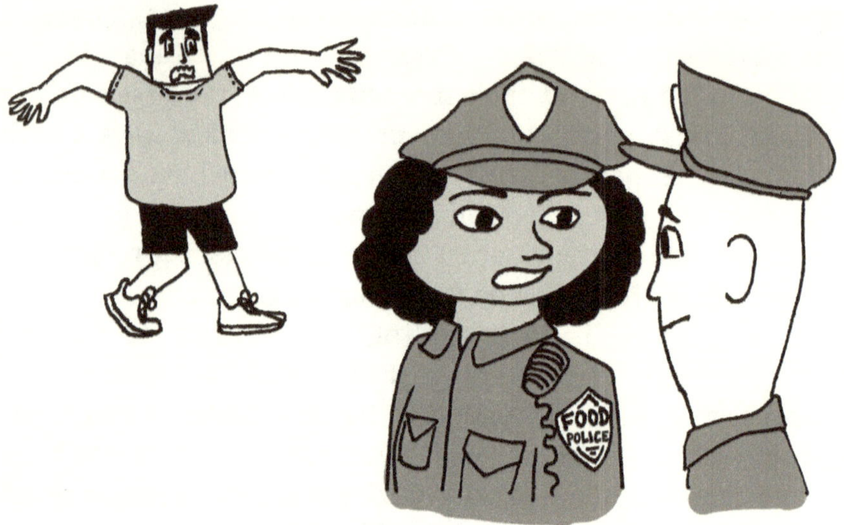

Cottage Cheese and Yogurt are tricky to classify because they often have sizable amounts of fat and carbs in them. If you are going to eat yogurt, just know that the flavored versions are dessert, not health food. Look at the macros for some of them. If you are going to get the pre-flavored yogurts, you might as well just stop pretending and enjoy some real ice cream. A better solution if you have a sweet craving would be to add in fresh fruit.

Also, if you are eating yogurt, have greek yogurt. It has a crazy amount more protein than normal yogurt, so is far superior. Greek yogurt actually tastes a lot like sour cream, and can be a great, healthy substitute for it in recipes. My parents have been tricking their dinner-party guests with greek yogurt instead of sour cream in their taco bar for years.

Cottage cheese also packs a great protein punch and can be worth eating if you enjoy the taste. It does have some fat and carbs in it, so be sure to mentally account for those. I love it with pepper sprinkled on top, but some people choose to go sweet and add fruit. A lot of old-school bodybuilders eat cottage cheese before bed because it has casein protein in it, which is slow digesting and digests all night so their bodies continue getting a steady stream of protein all night. For now, that is probably a small detail that doesn't really matter. The bottom line on cottage cheese and yogurt, like milk, is to enjoy them if you want, but be aware of their fat and carb contents and plan accordingly.

Supplements, in my opinion, are not necessary for weight loss. Many people have gotten very fit without them, and you can too. If you do include them within your diet, they should be a small, supplementary part of it, not a crucial piece. The problem is that if you get great results relying on supplements, you may feel the need to use them for the rest of your life, which goes against the entire point of building a multi-decade diet. I suggest that you focus on getting your diet right first, and if you still are interested in supplements later, use them in small quantities and see if you get results.

The list of supplements actually worth using is pretty short. Many are gimmicks or are built to make you feel like they work without actually giving you results. Most of the time, your best bet is to save your money for food or other things. However, there has been a lot of research, and I have had personal success with, whey protein, casein protein, and creatine.

Whey and casein are concentrated types of protein that are in milk, cottage cheese, and yogurt. The supplements just give you only the protein and not the other parts. I often take whey around workouts and casein before bed to get some extra protein in without having to cook additional food.

One of my favorite uses for whey is putting vanilla whey in milk with cereal. The additional protein makes the milk taste like vanilla ice cream, and turns the bowl of cereal into something that actually isn't nutritionally terrible. For those of you wondering, yes, I realize cereal has sugar in it and isn't that healthy, so if I am trying to get really lean, I reduce or remove cereal from my diet. Cereal aside, I've even gotten my supplement-hating dad to admit that milk with vanilla whey is amazing because while it tastes like a milkshake, it is actually relatively good for you.

If you do decide to use whey or casein supplements, do some research on the quality of them through lab testing web-sites such as labdoor.com, which checks for harmful substances and validates how much protein is actually in the supplements compared to what is on the label. If you can stand the taste, you are better off getting unflavored versions, or looking for ver-sions with the fewest added sweeteners.

Creatine is not caloric, but, at the highest level, helps the body process energy better so you can perform better athletic-ally. I think of it more of a sports-enhancing supplement than a weight loss supplement, and it can help you build more muscle. If you are more concerned about sports performance than just losing weight, consider looking into creatine, but know that it is by no means necessary. Before any gets up in arms, creatine is not a steroid, and is not banned for use by US college (NCAA) athletes, who have very strict doping standards.

There are dozens of other fat burners, muscle builders, and miscellaneous supplements out there. Many of them are either a huge waste of money, or are not sustainable over a lifetime. Some are dangerous and have been banned by some govern-ments. Do not worry that you are missing out by not using them. With them, as with all supplements, do your homework before you buy anything. Look for published research papers on their effects. See if NCAA athletes are allowed to take them. Consider how much they cost. Think about whether you could just improve your diet or you actually need these, or any, sup-plements.

Breakfast

You may also have noticed that breakfast as a whole hasn't

really been addressed by this chapter. That is because most of the "standard" breakfasts of pastries, cereal, and orange juice, although someone allowed them to be called "a balanced breakfast" on cereal boxes, are actually pretty bad for you. Most breakfasts are all carbs and sugar without much protein or nutrients to fill you up. There is not a separate category for breakfast. Not only that, but the American norm of having sweet things for breakfast is not universal. In Asia, many breakfasts are savory. Don't be fooled by the American breakfast, and don't be afraid to eat non "breakfast" foods in the morning.

If you still need something traditional or sweet for breakfast, a few principles will save you a lot of belly. Anchor your meal around protein-filled items like greek yogurt, eggs, and lean ham. Don't be afraid to add egg whites to your eggs if you want more protein. If you need sweets, have raw fruits rather than fruit juice or cereal. Try experimenting with smoothies - if created right and mostly comprised of healthy ingredients, they are not always unhealthy. Just beware of store-bought smoothies because many of those have added sugars in them.

Alcohol

I almost don't even want to touch alcohol as a subject because everyone has strong feelings about it. As of the writing of this book, the scientific community is in the middle of a heated debate on whether healthy levels of alcohol consumption exist. The debate will be long and drawn out because there are so many confounding variables to suss out.

As the science hopes to come to a verdict on alcohol that all sides are happy with, keep in mind that a lot of athletes don't drink in-season, and a lot of diet programs suggest no drinking. The verdict is far from in, but even so, everyone can agree that alcohol does have calories. Not only that, but if you are an athlete, it can slow your progress in two ways: drinking means your body stops protein synthesis, hampering muscle recovery[35], and it lowers your sleep quality[36], which is essential for recovery.

One telling fact about alcohol consumption: has your doctor ever told you to drink more to improve your health? If it was clearly and unambiguously good, doctors would tell non-drinkers to consider drinking. That hasn't happened.

With all that said, my recommendation on alcohol is to experiment and be aware that every drink does have calories in it. Some people quit drinking and lose a lot of weight quickly, and some quit drinking and are just sad. Know that the worst offenders from a body composition standpoint are calorie-rich full beers and sugar-heavy mixed drinks. Perhaps all you need to do is switch to either a light beer or a liquor you can drink with seltzer water or on the rocks. Don't worry, gentlemen, you don't have to have girly drinks: bourbon and scotch don't have added sugars.

If you are not seeing the results you want, try not drinking for a while and see if it makes a difference. Once you get the body you want, by all means, add the drinks back in. There is no booze ban here, just a warning to be aware that it can impact your results.

CHAPTER 15: NAVIGATING THE FOOD SPECTRUM

Now that you know what types of foods you are dealing with, let's return to the food spectrum and understand how it should be used. When you first look at it, you are probably thinking, "crap, I have to eat just meat and veggies the rest of my life?" the answer is unequivocally NO!

1	2	3	4	5	6	7	8	9
Lean meat, veggies	Lean meat, veggies, complex carbs	Lean meat, veggies, complex carbs, nuts	Fatty meat, veggies, complex carbs	Fatty meat, complex carbs	Fried meats	(Fried) savory nonmeats	Desserts	Sugary drinks
Healthiest								Unhealthiest

In fact, levels 1 (lean meat and veggies only) and 2 (lean meat, veggies, and complex carbs only) don't need to be your full main diet at all. You can live a very lean, healthy life mostly in the 3 (lean meat, veggies, complex carbs, nuts) to 4 (fatty meat, veggies, complex carbs) range. If you decide you want to get even leaner and into the fitness model range, you'll need to spend more time in 1 and 2, but for just normal weight loss you can usually stay in the 3 to 4 range and do just fine.

The magic of this spectrum is the endless number of possibilities and the combinations you can, and more realistically, will, have to create with it. Given how everyone's body is unique and influenced by activity levels and the order they eat things, it isn't as simple as saying box 1 plus box 7 equals box 4, but there are ways you can play both sides of the spectrum to your advantage.

Since this system is built on sustainability, I am not going to tell you to immediately go to box number 3. In fact, especially if you are far over on the right side of the spectrum, immediately going to 3 is the worst thing you can do. You want to do the least amount of work to have the most amount of change. This is something that author Tim Ferriss talks about a lot, the minimum effective dose ("MED"): the smallest dose that will produce a desired outcome. In this framework, anything beyond the MED is wasteful.

What this means for dieting is that if there are 10 steps to the perfect diet, you just want to take the first one, because if you take all ten at once, you have no more changes to make if that doesn't work. Don't eat like a fitness model yet, just eat like a slightly skinnier version of your current self.

Before we go into how a hypothetical dieter would go from box 9 to box 3, let me reiterate: the key is simplicity and hitting the low-hanging fruit.

One of my friends in school ended up losing around 30 pounds one semester. He had been asking me all kinds of nutrition and exercise advice, and I felt like I had been letting him down because I never had amazing answers for him. I didn't see him for a few months, and then one day we ran into each other. He looked like a different person. I remember asking him what he'd done.

"Honestly, I just stopped eating so much crap. I cut out cookies, and the pounds came right off."

We aren't all as lucky as he was to know exactly what is keeping us heavier than we want to be, but if you are, take advantage! You are very fortunate if you know exactly what is making you fatter than you want to be and can just eliminate it. If you have obviously too many sugary drinks and desserts, axing those alone may do the trick. However, the key is making it stick without feeling like you are depriving yourself. The way to do that is with moderation and a gradual approach.

People are smart. They usually know what is healthy and what isn't. The problem isn't knowledge, it is behavioral change. If you go too fast, you risk making it so painful that you rebound back to right where you were. Now, let's talk through a hypothetical person going from boxes 8 and 9 to 3 and 4.

Let's say you subsist entirely in boxes 8 and 9, on sugary drinks and desserts. If you do what many dieters do and jump headlong into box 1, only eating lean meat and veggies, a lot of bad things may happen.

Jumping directly into box 1 would cause your calories to drop dramatically, unless you manage to eat as many calories eating meat and veggies as you could with desserts, which would be very difficult to do. This would likely lead to huge cravings. Soon you likely would be unable to stop yourself from going back to your old diet of desserts and sugary drinks, and you would be right back where you started.

You will not only feel like a huge failure, but you will be upset by how hard it was to resist your cravings. You may never want to diet again, and may be convinced that dieting is something that only a fortunate few can successfully do. You'll find statistics on how the majority of diets fail and conclude that you can never change.

I firmly believe that most diets fail because people are doing the wrong ones, or are doing the right ones but doing them incorrectly.

While dropping directly into box 1 and cutting your calories rapidly may seem very effective at first, it is so drastic that your body may freak out and react against it. If this happens, and for some reason you don't actually lose weight with your drastic shift into box 1, you will have no more changes to make since your calories are already so low and you are already eating only meat and veggies. If you want to go any further, you have to resort to unconventional measures, like a juice cleanse or fat loss supplements. If you want your diet to succeed, be patient and move slow enough that you keep some bullets in your arsenal if you aren't making progress.

Therefore, a more effective, sustainable, and enjoyable approach would be to slowly migrate left on the scale. If you started in boxes 8 and 9, you would first aim to live in boxes 7 and 8, slowly replacing some of your sugary drinks with (fried) savory non-meats. This would likely have a small impact, but at least you would be chewing more calories, which might fill you up a bit longer. You would keep doing this until you stopped losing weight.

This way, you are making tiny changes that are not painful. You're replacing soda with french fries - not exactly herculean. You would milk that for as long as you could, getting your body used to the new diet, until you stopped losing weight.

Then, when you stall, you would venture into box 6, having fried meats instead of fried non-meats, adding a bit more protein into your diet instead of sugary items, slowly moving along the spectrum with the majority of your calories now coming from boxes 6 and 7 instead of 8 and 9. You would continue to enjoy this until your weight stopped dropping.

Once you stall again, you'd venture into box 5, which has two big changes. It is fatty non-fried meats, which removes the extra calories caused by frying, and complex carbohydrates, which are healthier than the majority of the (fried) savory non-meats. This really means replacing chips or fries with rice, grain or fruit. At this point, you'd be almost entirely off of dessert and sugary drinks and eating the majority of your food with meat and real carbohydrates in it.

When you are ready to make another move, the jump to box 4 is a big one because it introduces one of the most important elements in your arsenal: vegetables! Everyone knows that "you should eat your vegetables", but they are portrayed as a boring thing that just your mother wants you to do. However, Popeye had it right. Veggies are the key to success. As mentioned before, they fill you up but have a minimum of calories.

You can literally eat veggies all day if you want and not gain weight, as long as you haven't drowned them in butter, oil, or cheese. If you are trying to lose weight, you should become best friends with vegetables. Keep that stomach so busy and distracted digesting broccoli that it couldn't dream of having another bite of anything else. Also, in addition to keeping your immune system going, veggies are full of nutrients that improve your hormone patterns, increasing your testosterone levels which make you build muscle and lose fat faster.

Getting to box 4 is key. Once you've got veggies in your diet, you're really in business.

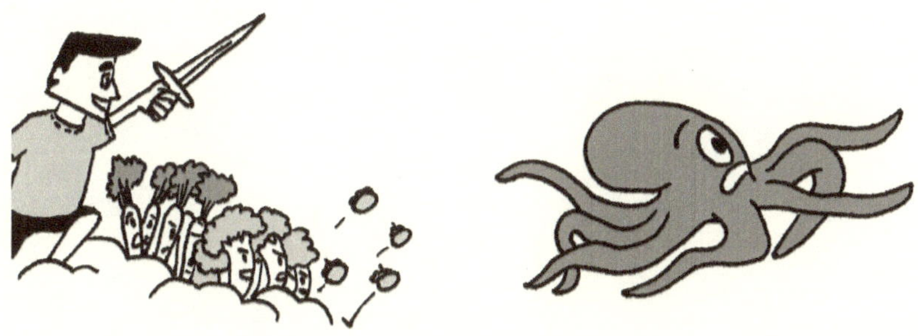

The final tweak, as you move to box 3, is replacing your fatty meats with lean meats and nuts. Now, before you get all up in arms, you don't have to always eat lean meats, and there are some great fatty meats which we have already discussed. However, lean meats bring a few benefits. Since lean meats have hardly any fat in them, you will need to get your fat from nuts (as mentioned, we are also classifying avocados in the "nuts" category). This is a better way to do it because nuts have fiber that the meat fat does not, meaning they will fill you up even more, and nuts have more monounsaturated and polyunsaturated fats, which doctors are convinced are better for your heart than other types of fats[37].

The other angle to nuts, which we've mentioned before, is

that they allow you more flexibility than fatty meats to adapt for unexpected fatty foods. If you accidentally have a fatty meal, you can just remove nuts from your next meal to compensate. This is far easier than trying to get the fat out of fatty meat.

Here you are, living in box 3 (lean meats, veggies, complex carbs, and nuts) as your home base, with quick trips to the other boxes as needed. If you get here and stay here for a few months, you will likely see a huge improvement in your body composition. At some point, you will plateau, and you will need to think about changing portion sizes and going into other boxes strategically, which is what our next chapters will cover.

CHAPTER 16: HOW MUCH TO EAT

◆ ◆ ◆

It was my sophomore year of college, and I had my diet and lifting dialed in. Every meal was planned to the minute, and I was hitting personal records in the gym left and right. Except one week, I screwed up.

In the two water bottle holders on my backpack: one always contained my water bottle, and the other kept a container of peanuts that I would use to add some extra calories into my afternoon meals. Every Sunday, I would go to the grocery store and get a new one pound container of peanuts, along with my other regular groceries.

One week I forgot the peanuts.

The store wasn't that far away, but between exams, social events, my part-time job, and extracurriculars, I didn't have a spare minute to go get more peanuts. In the frenzy of college life, I quickly forgot about them.

At the end of the week, something weird happened. I was getting dressed and found that my belt had stretched out - it was about an inch too loose for me to fit, even looped through the last hole. Frustrated, I decided I would go without the belt. Yet my pants were too big, and were so loose that they were falling off. It didn't make any sense.

I went to the scale and weighed myself. I was down 5 pounds, and hadn't even realized it. My energy levels hadn't changed. The only thing different was the peanuts. I was just having less total calories, and it made a dramatic change.

I share this story not because I don't like peanuts - they are awesome - but to illustrate how even if your diet is otherwise perfect, if you are eating too many calories, you will weigh too much. Moving to the right spot on the food spectrum is helpful, but even when you are doing that, at some point you will simply have to eat less if you want to make more progress. This chapter is here to help you figure out how much to eat and how to determine relative portions of what you eat.

So far in the book, I've been intentionally vague on portion sizes to account for differences in people's own size and diet style. There are multiple ways to skin a cat, and you don't have to measure everything to the tenth degree. However, as a general rule, once you get to box 3 (lean protein, vegetables, complex carbs, nuts) and stay there for a few months, you are likely already close to your ideal weight, but a little bit heavier than you want.

This is where it gets frustrating for many people. To get that last level of leanness, you will have to cut your portions. There isn't an exact amount here, because there are dozens of confounding variables. The only right answer is that you need to eat less than you do now. It's not rocket science.

Directionally, you should have the most veggies, a smaller amount of meat and carbs, and the smallest amount of nuts. In proportions, this may look like 40% veggies, 25% meat, 25% carbs, and 10% nuts, but you can ratchet up the veggies if desired.

I hesitate with giving exact portion sizes because there is so much disagreement among people. Let's start with the one that will likely change the least as you vary phases of your diet: protein. Some people swear by getting 1 gram per pound of bodyweight per day. Others insist you only need 1 gram per pound of lean body mass, while others say you can get by on 0.8 grams per pound if you are an athlete. You could spend the rest of your life researching it. Before we get to an exact amount, a few things to know about protein.

Protein is one of the body's building blocks. If you don't have any in your diet, you'll fall apart. Even vegetarians and vegans admit this and spend a lot of time making sure they have enough protein in their diet. You can cut out carbs, or fats, and be ok, but cutting out protein will have the most deleterious impact on your health.

Protein is very filling and curbs cravings. You may have noticed a lot of food items have recently been advertising how their protein content is. The public has finally caught on to the fact that protein can control appetite, and food producers are milking it for all its worth.

In addition, protein will help you recover, build, and maintain muscle. It comes especially in handy as you lose weight, as protein helps you maintain your muscle mass as you lose fat, so that once you finally shed all that fat you won't just look like a sad skeleton. Some diets will even say to increase your protein when you are losing weight for this reason.

Given those three points, it should be clear that protein is good for you. So how much should you have?

I don't like laying stakes in the sand, but am going to recommend 1 gram per pound of bodyweight. Depending on your bodyweight, that is likely a pound or more of meat per day. You're going to have to learn to cook that. Yes, that is higher than some minimum recommendations, but remember, those are minimums. We are looking for the maximum benefit and trying to take advantage of the filling and any muscle-related benefits we can get from protein. It gives you a good amount of filling calories and will help you steer clear of too many un-filling and fattening foods.

So why not more protein? Few people recommend above 1 gram per pound of bodyweight, simply because studies haven't found additional benefit from it. Additional grams of protein mean less fat and carbs in your diet, because if you have a constant amount of calories, the remainder has to come from somewhere. You might as well enjoy the rest of your calories more than you would pure meat. Also, if you are an athlete or exercising, you'll benefit from the energy boost from some carbohydrates in your diet that you will have space for without extra protein.

Finally, and most practically for a lot of people, protein is expensive and can be a pain to prepare. Save yourself the money and the time and don't aim for more than 1 gram per day.

As far as amounts of carbs and fats go, this will vary. If you want to do a low carb or low fat diet, be my guest. What I've found over the years is that you can do those and they work fine, but no better than a balanced diet with controlled amounts of calories. Having about a third of your calories from carbs, a third from fats, and a third from protein will probably work for most people to get them to very respectable levels of leanness.

Note that fats have 9 calories per gram while proteins and carbs have 4, so a gram of fat has about twice the calories of the other two. This means that 20 grams of fat is more like 45 grams of protein or carbs, from a calorie perspective. As far as exact proportions, a few percentage points here and there don't really matter that much.

Play around with your fats and carbs and see what happens, but make sure your protein stays constant and your total calories stay constant. Keep the veggie portions big as they are a great filler, or even consider adding more veggies as you lower portions of other things to keep you full. You may find that your body reacts a lot better to things on one end or the other. Generally, if you are exercising more, you'll want to have relatively more carbs as they will improve your performance and make you feel less tired. Specifically, you'll want to have more carbs on exercise days and less on non-exercise days.

When you decide you need to lose more weight, lower your carbs or fats a little bit and keep them at this lower level for a week. See what happens. If you lose over a half pound that week, maintain the lower level for of carbs or fats for another week until you don't lose any weight. When you don't lose any weight, lower your fats or carbs again by a little bit and maintain for a week. Rinse and repeat.

This should not be traumatic, because you are just eating a little bit less of the same thing. This is having three quarters of a cup of rice instead of a full cup, or two tablespoons of nuts instead of three. It should be very low drama. That is the idea.

This may sound too simple, and you may be upset I am not giving an exact amount or ratio to eat. That isn't necessary, because you are not a robot and don't need every ounce of food that goes into you weighed down to the gram. More than that, the more precision you add in, the more difficult it will be to keep your diet "under control", and the more painful it will be to do for decades. You can skip the precision but if you are directionally right and consistent for weeks at a time, the right things will happen. You've got a life to live - stop worrying so much about the minutiae!

If you do want to worry about the minutiae, there are lots of great apps and programs that can tell you the calories and macros in everything. However, just know that until you are either a competitive athlete or down to very low levels of body fat, simply eyeballing things and consistently lowering portions will get you 90% of the results with a lot less effort. It likely isn't worth your time until you get very lean.

Now I'll turn it over to my Dad, who will share his specific meals. Keep in mind that these are the portions that work for him with his height, weight, age, and activity levels. They won't be the same as yours, but they should give you an understanding of general principles and how important portions are.

Mark here - You just read quite a bit about what and how to eat from Henry. We mostly agree, but I wanted to share my ideas from my own perspective.

I'm hoping that you are still reading along and that you have embraced the right weight target for yourself. Now that you've recovered from that shock, I risk giving you another shock by telling you how much, or how little you can eat.

Let's talk about calories. Calories are a unit of energy. In the scientific sense, a calorie is the amount of heat energy required to raise one gram of water by one degree celsius at an atmospheric pressure equal to one. Ok, forget the science. As it relates to food and weight, calories are a measure of the stored energy (fuel) in the foods that you eat. Calories consumed in food provide the energy that you need to survive.

Let me say it right now: a calorie is a calorie. A calorie from a donut provides the same amount of fuel for your body as a calorie from a chicken breast. I am not suggesting that you go on a donut diet, but you could and would lose weight if you eat fewer donut calories than your body uses. There are lots of reasons to avoid the donut-only diet, which I mentioned in the "What to Eat" chapter.

If you consume fewer calories than your body burns, you will lose weight. If you consume more calories than your body burns, you will gain weight. I know that is simple and obvious, so remember it and live by it. There are no magic foods that by themselves cause you to lose weight.

To find out the right calorie count for yourself, start with your Basal Metabolic Rate ("BMR"). Simply stated, this is the amount of calories that you consume by existing and not exercising. There are numerous free calculators available online that will calculate your BMR based on inputs of your height, weight, and age. Remember that you will need to use your goal weight to determine your target BMR calories. If you are 30 lbs overweight, your BMR will be higher. Get ready for another shock. Your BMR calories are pretty low. See the two examples below:

5' 10" Male age 45 targeting a healthy weight of 153 lbs at BMI of 22. BMR Calories per day = 1585

5'4" Female age 45 targeting a healthy weight of 122 lbs at a BMI of 21. BMR Calories per day = 1183

Let's assume for the moment that you are mostly sedentary. If you are currently above your target weight, you will have to consume your target BMR calories or fewer to reach your target weight. The further below your BMR calories you consume, the faster you will lose weight.

Hopefully you aren't sedentary and you are burning some additional calories, but even if you consider yourself fairly active, it probably isn't that many calories. If you exercise 1-3 times per week, and walk a good bit, you are probably burning an additional 400 calories per day. If you use a fitness tracker or a smart watch, you likely have more accurate data. Let's keep it simple and assume you are burning an additional 400 calories a day, which you can add to your BMR calorie allotment. Unless you are really tall, you just learned that to lose weight you need to consume under 2000 calories per day, and maybe a lot less than 2000! Sorry.

If you eat to your BMR + Exercise caloric allotment, you will achieve your target weight over time. It really is just math. However, it will take too long. Eat about 1200 calories a day and you will lose the weight very quickly. I know this sounds horrible, but you will enjoy the reward of shedding those pounds quickly.

Adhering to portion size is absolutely critical to success. The good news is that calories per portion size are available on almost all foods and there are numerous online calorie guides that will give you calories per ounce of almost any food you can think of. The bad news is that appropriate portion sizes are pretty small. At first, you will be shocked when you put a four ounce portion of meat on your plate. You can eat large portions of most vegetables as long as you don't cover them in a caloric sauce. Breads and grains have to be eaten in quite small quantities.

Here is an example of what I ate while trying to lose weight quickly:

Breakfast:
1 egg fried in less than 1 teaspoon of olive oil - ~100 calories
1 oz. slice of organic ham - ~35 calories
1 slice of light 5 grain toast - ~75 calories
3 oz. whole milk in numerous cups of coffee ~50 calories
For a total of 260 calories I eat a breakfast that fills me and keeps me full until lunchtime.

Lunch:
1 bag tuna - ~ 90 calories
1 oz cheese - ~80 calories (for white cheese like feta or goat)
6 whole wheat crackers ~ 120 calories

A small handful of berries ~40 calories

Water or calorie free sparkling water

The above provides a satisfying lunch for 330 calories. You can substitute some of the above with a cup of plain yogurt, a few olives, or a couple of very small slices of dried meat. Lately, I've been replacing the lunch items with a Spinach / Blueberry protein smoothie.

Dinner:

So far, if you didn't snack, you've eaten less than 600 calories. That leaves you 400 - 600 for dinner. I suggest the following:

4 oz portion of meat ~ 150-200 calories

Large portion of vegetables (try seasoning with plain mustard or lemon juice.) ~80 calories

1 measured portion of beans, potatoes, rice or other grain, small amount of oil or butter ~ 150 calories.

Water or calorie-free sparkling water

Total calories ~ 430.

All in you've consumed about 1100 calories. You can probably add a glass or two of red wine for 150-300 calories and be at a 1400 grand total. If you do this 6 days a week, you will lose weight. Quickly. You can have a "cheat" day once a week without doing much harm.

Henry here - Finding your BMR is incredibly important. Maybe you don't track your calories every day - that is fine. However, it is an incredibly important exercise to find your BMR, since it is probably a lot lower than you'd think. The 2,000 calorie a day guideline is, like most averages, totally unrepresentative of most people. Don't assume that 2,000 is your number, or more importantly, a fair number.

There is no fairness in dieting. Your body doesn't care what number you have in your head. It just cares about how much energy it needs to maintain weight. If you give it more calories than that number, you will gain weight, and your body will continue not caring. If you give it less calories than that number, you will lose weight. Simple as that.

Also, you'll notice that Mark's recommendation of 1,200 calories is around a 25% calorie cut, more dramatic than the 15%

drops I've mentioned elsewhere. That worked for him. It may work for you, it may not. It is a bit more dramatic than I am comfortable with, but most importantly, it is not halving your calories, just cutting them by a quarter. If you find it is too dramatic and you are yo-yoing back up, maybe try a 15% or 20% calorie cut.

If you want to count calories on a regular basis like he does, go for it. My approach is a little different: instead of counting actual calories, I just focus on portion sizes, and keep them relatively constant, decreasing when I want to lose weight. This is less precise, but directionally accurate and simple enough for me to not mind doing it, so works over time. Finally, I wholeheartedly disagree with my Dad's propensity to stick with the single meat portion sizes. I think you should size your own meat portions by dividing up your protein allotment and cutting from there, and that he doesn't eat enough protein.

However, his main message - portion sizes are important - is something nobody can escape from.

CHAPTER 17: REQUIRED VS EXTRACURRICULAR EATING

◆ ◆ ◆

One of the great mysteries of my adult life has been why I don't actually crave unhealthy foods the way most people do, and when I do eat them, why I never go wild and eat too much of them. At times it has been awkward when people have told me "I wish I had your willpower," but I've always known it wasn't willpower. It was something else that I couldn't put my finger on.

Recently, the answer has become more clear: I prioritize my eating. Even more important than which foods you eat is the order in which you eat them.

Priorities matter because everything you eat fills your stomach up and makes you less hungry. Things farther on the left of the food spectrum, below, fill you up more with less calories.

So let's make things easy. Avoid 9 (sugary drinks) because they are terrible, but everything else on the spectrum is fair game, with one catch: after you get your fill from the first box on the spectrum. You can eat your French fries, but only after you are filled up on lean meat and veggies.

1	2	3	4	5	6	7	8	9
Lean meat, veggies	Lean meat, veggies, complex carbs	Lean meat, veggies, complex carbs, nuts	Fatty meat, veggies, complex carbs	Fatty meat, complex carbs	Fried meats	(Fried) savory nonmeats	Desserts	Sugary drinks

Healthiest   Unhealthiest

I call this required vs. extracurricular eating. The veggies and lean meats are required. They fill you up and keep your body in top shape. Once you finish eating them for the day, if you must, you can venture into extracurriculars: the middle or right side of the spectrum.

Now this seems obvious, but it really makes an impact in situations where you are going to be tempted by delicious and unhealthy foods.

Imagine your most indulgent food fantasy. Waiters are walking around with all the foods you dream about. Now imagine you have to eat a plate of veggies and chicken first, and then you can go eat all your fantasy foods. Odds are that you will eat a lot less of the fantasy food since you are already full of chicken and veggies.

Maybe your zeal to eat the fantasy food doesn't get dimmed by the chicken and veggies. That's great, but your stomach will still be filled up with it, so you physically don't have space to eat as much as you might have of the fantasy food.

Moving into a more realistic situation, notice that I said the veggies and lean meats are required. Generally, I'd recommend nuts and complex carbs as well, but you can skip those if you know you have a big dinner coming up, knowing that you will get plenty of carbs and fats at the dinner.

By eating the veggies and lean meats first, not only will you eat a bit less at dinner because you're already filled up, but you do get to enjoy tasty foods without going totally overboard on the calories since you won't be ravenous. Congratulations, you have tricked your body! Now let's do it consistently and watch the results slowly roll in.

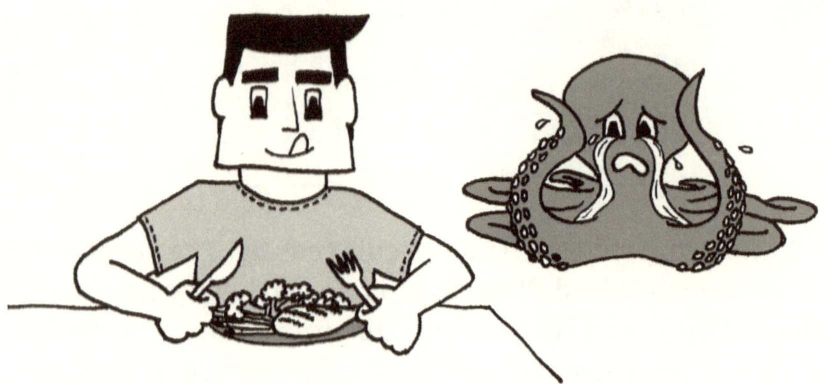

I use this sometimes if there is a birthday party or some-where I want to eat cake or similarly unhealthy foods. I skip the rice and nuts I usually have with my lunch, so I have a deficit of carbs and fats in my day. When cake time comes around, I get to indulge without feeling guilty. The best part? Not feeling like a robot who never eats sugar.

This will make a big impact psychologically and may be the difference between adhering to a diet and deciding you just aren't a "dieting person". You aren't saying you can't eat the des-sert, just saying you have to eat your broccoli and chicken first. But wait - here's the best part: after you eat the broccoli and chicken, you either don't want the dessert at all, or end up eat-ing a lot less of it.

If the required vs extracurricular working isn't working for you, try adding more veggies to your required eating before you can eat your extracurriculars. If you do it right, at some point, the sheer quantity of veggies becomes exhausting and eating becomes a chore. By the time you finish your required eating, the thought of eating anything else is almost repulsive, and you would rather skip the dessert altogether for a reprieve from chewing. Your stomach will be so full, and your jaw so tired of chewing, that you will want nothing to do with additional food. People will look at you like you are a total nut for not craving the cake in front of you, but you will not be interested. The exact amount of veggies to eat will vary on what you are used to and your size, but to give you an idea, I eat at minimum about a pound of veggies per day, and increase the amount if I'm trying and struggling to lose weight. Gotta keep that stomach full!

I call this concept "pre-eating" and have used it many times to both achieve better dieting outcomes and to save money at restaurants. Right before going out to dinner, I'll eat a big chicken breast and bowl of veggies. I'll be stuffed at the table and usually end up ordering something small and reasonable. This is a diet-saver if you are about to go out for something indulgent like pizza or pasta, dramatically cutting down how much you'll end up eating.

Ironically, I started doing this not as a calorie-reduction mechanism, but because so many restaurants in New York have small portion sizes and I didn't want to have to order two entrees to actually get full.

If you feel like a child having your parents tell you "you can have your ice cream after you eat your vegetables" you're right, because that is exactly what is happening. The wisdom of eating dessert after dinner brilliantly takes advantage of the physiology we've just outlined above, and has been used to keep people from eating too much dessert for centuries.

To be clear, this is not a suggestion to not eat anything other than lean meat and veggies. It is just a suggestion that you make sure you hit your thresholds on those foods, and are flexible with your fats and carbs in case you need to use them for "extra-curricular" aka fun eating. If there is no cake in your future, you still benefit from eating your normal amount of carbs and fats. Carbs and fats are energy, and important to eat, because if you don't eat them at all, you may lose weight, but you will likely awaken terrible cravings.

Cravings

Cravings are everyone's favorite diet de-railer. Weirdly, I didn't really have them much until I gained weight on my "bulk" described in the introduction, but as I got fatter, I craved more and more unhealthy foods. Then, when I lost the weight, strangely, the cravings magically went away. That was my first hint that cravings are not necessarily an unavoidable thing. Over the years, I have noticed cravings come and go, with a few trends: when I get fatter, the cravings come back. They also come back when I am dramatically under-cutting my calories.

Tying this back to earlier in the book, the cravings are strongest when I am too far in either direction on the fat and happy scale. If you try to lose weight too fast by dramatically cutting calories, you are probably about to get a whole mess of cravings. Not only that, but some cravings are caused by thirst or lack of nutrients - they are your body trying to tell you something, not a sign of mental weakness.

The ultimate tragedy is an obese person who is malnourished but constantly craving more food because their body is hoping for nutrients, but only gets fat and carbs from the unhealthy foods they eat, leaving the body to create even more cravings. They are simultaneously starving and getting fatter. The idea of extracurricular eating is to make sure that your cravings are not just malnutrition or pure hunger in disguise.

The rabbit hole goes a little deeper. Eating speed and digestion speed make an impact on how fattening your meals are. This is pretty well studied, with conclusions that "eating slower inhibited the development of obesity[38]" and that "slow spaced eating may be a useful prevention strategy, but might also help curb food intake in those already suffering from obesity and diabetes[39]." So if you are going to eat dessert or unhealthy foods, do yourself a favor and eat it very slowly. Enjoy every bite instead of just inhaling it.

That is the key to required vs. extracurricular eating: only eat unhealthy foods when you are already full of healthy ones, and you are forced to eat them slower.

This all comes back to insulin that we've talked about before. When you eat anything, your body releases insulin that signals that there is sugar coming into the bloodstream that needs to be used by the cells. When you eat something like a vegetable, which is made of very complex molecules, your body has to break it down into little pieces before it can turn into glucose to be absorbed by the cells, which takes time.

Compare this to eating sugar, which is already broken down and can be absorbed by the cells immediately. With the vegetable, since it takes some time to digest, your body can release the right amount of insulin and all the nutrients can be absorbed by the cells. However, with the sugar, if you eat a lot of it, it will come into your bloodstream so fast that your body can't release enough insulin fast enough for your cells to absorb it all for energy. The excess becomes stored as body fat, and you get fatter.

In other words, there are two variables here: eating speed and the complexity of food you eat. Maybe you can't avoid eating sugar, but you can at least do it slowly so your body has time to digest it and not just store it as fat. By consuming the sugar more slowly, your body won't have to release as much insulin, and you will be less likely to suffer from the effects of high blood sugar (in the short-term that is tiredness, which is where the term "food coma" comes from).

Implementing Required vs Extracurricular Eating

If you really want to make this stick, you are going to have to make it as easy as possible to keep required foods on hand and to make extracurricular foods hard to get. For required foods, make sure you keep them regularly stocked, or consider ordering your groceries online. Especially if you are the type of person who often gets distracted in grocery stores and fills up your cart with unnecessary treats, this may help a lot. The beauty of ordering groceries online is that many services have an option to make the delivery recurring, so you don't even have to think and you will always have a steady supply of healthy foods around. If you are not into online ordering, you will have to be vigilant at the grocery store.

Grocery stores are treacherous places, full of overpriced junk food and junk food masquerading as health food. The junk food is usually obviously unhealthy, but beware. First, advertisers will milk any health angle they can, advertising things like "fat free" on candy that is pure sugar, or "now with less sugar" on something that now has less sugar but double the fat. Not only that, but most of the junk food you'll see is a huge waste of money for the nutrients and even pure calories you are getting.

Let's bring this home and talk about something you have probably tried before: potato chips. As of the time this book was written, for $2.48, you can get an 8 oz bag of brand name potato chips online, which has 8 servings for a total of 120 grams of carbs, 80 grams of fat, 16 grams of protein, and 1,280 calories.

This means a dollar of potato chips gets you approximately 516 calories, 48 grams of carbs, 32 grams of fat, and 6 grams of protein.

Now let's compare to a bag of rice, and we'll even get the fancy, good stuff: jasmine rice, in a small bag which costs more because you are not buying in bulk. For $5.68 also online, you can get a 5 pound bag of jasmine rice, which has 1,890 grams of carbs, 0 grams of fat, 135 grams of protein, and 8,100 calories. This means a dollar gets you approximately 1,426 calories, 333 grams of carbs, 0 grams of fat, and 26 grams of protein.

That means that a dollar of rice gets you nearly triple the calories that a dollar of potato chips gets you.

Now of course your reaction is that potato chips are so much better than rice, and have a lot more fat that is delicious and keeps you full.

Ok, I'll play ball.

Let's get some salted cocktail peanuts to go with our rice to add a crunch, some fat, and some salt. For $2.48, the exact same price of the chips, you can get a 1 pound can of cocktail peanuts which has 16 servings for a total of 64 grams of carbs, 240 grams of fat, 128 grams of protein, and 2,720 calories. Per dollar, this is 1,097 calories, 26 grams of carbs, 97 grams of fat, and 52 grams of protein. Even the peanuts are twice the calories per dollar of potato chips.

Let's tie it all together. You've got $10 and decide to spend it on either rice and peanuts or potato chips. You buy 4 bags of chips for $9.92, and get 516 calories per dollar. Or, you can buy 1 bag of rice and 2 things of peanuts for $10.64, and get 1,273 calories per dollar. Your call.

Assume we were really trying to pinch pennies and wanted to get cheaper, less tasty rice, buying a 20 pound bag of rice for $9.96. You'd get 3,042 calories per dollar. Spend a minute looking at the table below to see just how expensive that cheap bag of potato chips is compared to some basics:

Item	Cost	Cals/$	Carb/$	Fat/$	Pro/$
20lb Rice	$9.96	3,042	710	0	61
5lb Jasmine Rice	$5.68	1,426	333	0	26
$10 Rice + Peanuts	$10.64	1,273	190	45	38
Peanuts	$2.48	1,097	26	97	52
Potato Chips	$2.48	516	48	32	6

Concerns about lack of nutrients and protein aside, rice is unbelievably cheap. You wouldn't be that healthy, but if you found a way to cook it, you could live on a dollar of food a day by just eating rice, even in the United States. If you wanted to actually nourish yourself, you could eat a pound of chicken breast ($3), a pound of frozen veggies ($3), a few servings of rice ($1), and a few servings of peanuts ($1) and get a full day's food for $8.

Stop pretending basic food is that expensive. The marked up, deliciously flavored stuff is, because they are doing the work of making it tasty and packaging it for you. It is your money, and you can choose to spend it how you want, just know that when you buy most junk food you are lining the pockets of the food industry.

Now the other, more sinister side of the spectrum of expensive junk food is expensive health food that is actually junk food in disguise. I don't care if your cookies are organic and made with natural cane sugar - they are still full of sugar. I don't care that you are drinking 100% fruit juice full of vitamins - it is still fruit juice with all the sugar and none of the beneficial, filling fiber of raw fruit. Those dried fruits you love so much have less nutrients and are far more calorically dense than their raw, water-filled cousins. That granola bar with "extra protein" is still mostly just carbs and fat. The healthy cereal with oats and nuts in it has twice the calories per cup of many of the sugary types.

You could spend an entire lifetime finding bogus "health" foods in grocery stores. While some really are good for you, there are also dozens that are just as bad as the cookies you really want to eat. Pay attention to the nutrition facts - you may be surprised. Know that many will be healthy-ish: healthier than the really indulgent normal edition, but only marginally so, and often with a higher price tag attached. Always be skeptical.

With this in mind, you need to go into grocery stores ready for hand to hand combat.

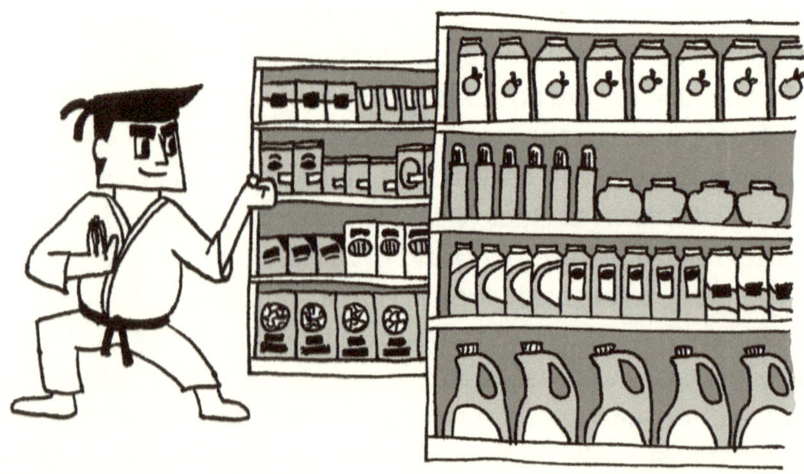

You are going to be tempted by those tasty little artisan cookies, and the kale chips that seem so healthy and may taste almost as good as the sour cream and onion chips you really want. You need to stay strong and don't give in. Don't spend your precious money on things your body doesn't need and will just make you fat. If you can shut the food down now, you spare your future self from having to say no when it is sitting on your counter at home, free for the taking. There is a barrier to entry now: the price of buying it. Resist - you can do it!

It really does help to follow the common wisdom of not shopping while hungry and going in with a list knowing exactly what you want. As mentioned, if you happen to live somewhere that has a grocery delivery service, it can sometimes be worth the money and convenience to get your food delivered, with the added benefit of having no surprise purchases if you set your order to just repeat every week.

Empty the Pantry

Now, you've dodged the junk food and gotten the groceries you need. Great work. But if you are like most people, you probably have a secret stash of cookies, candy, or chips somewhere. Throw these extracurricular foods out. Now. The trash police aren't going to come and shame you for wasting perfectly good junk food. You've already paid for it with your money, and you can either pay for it with your health or get rid of it. You need to get over your guilt for wasting things. Learning to trash unhealthy foods will pay dividends for your entire life. You should not have bought them in the first place, and eating them instead of trashing them may make you feel better mentally, but is slowing your progress.

You do not get a medal of honor for eating half a cookie instead of throwing it away, you just get a gut.

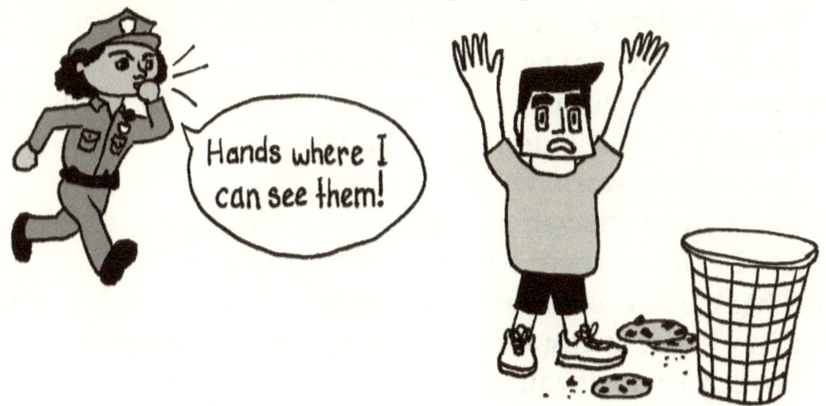

Keeping unhealthy foods around just adds to temptation. You aren't weak for not being able to resist the cookies in your pantry. Few people can resist such easily accessible, tasty delights. You are weak for keeping them around as a backup. This isn't the apocalypse - you don't need cookies to eat when the zombies come. You need cheap peanuts. Stop pretending you need junk food around.

Your goal is to create a barrier to entry, so if you really want those cookies, you have to work for them and go to the store and get them specifically. Implement the plan we discussed in the "Start with Soda" chapter with any other type of junk food you are craving, which will save you from eating it just because it was there and seemed good at the time. Actually tasting the food will mean so much more after making the journey to the store if you really want it.

If you can make it as hard as possible to get these things, then statistically, you will eat less of them. In a moment of weakness when you decide to eat cookies, if you have to actually have them, make a trip to the store to get them. The additional effort of actually having to go to the store just for the cookies means that you are simply less likely to go. Don't forget that your body wants to be lazy if you'll let it.

Use this laziness to your advantage, and don't waste your willpower trying not to eat junk food in your pantry - just don't buy it in the first place.

If you do decide you really need the cookies, buy them at the store, eat what you need, and throw the rest away or donate them to a food pantry or to someone in need. If this is hard for you, maybe you shouldn't have bought them in the first place. Either way, the world will go on.

Also consider never buying sweets at the grocery store at all and only having them a la carte at restaurants. This gives you another barrier to entry: usually they cost more per bite when you buy them at restaurants, giving you even more incentive to not buy them. If you do end up ordering dessert, you usually get a single serving of it, not the entire cake, so you don't have to feel guilty for throwing away the rest. If you want two slices, you have to order another full order, instead of just walking back into the kitchen and cutting yourself another slice.

Navigating Social Settings

Mark here - Eating is a very social activity. Eating the way that I described in "What to Eat" is reasonably easy when you are at home. Eating light at work and in social settings is very hard. Your well-meaning friends may even try to ambush you!

Restaurants are a real challenge. There is a reason most everything tastes good - all that butter and salt!

First, avoiding eating breakfast out. A big carb and calorie load is a bad way to start your day. Eat breakfast at home, if you don't have time to cook, try having a boiled egg and a small cup of plain yogurt. A note on the yogurt.

If you add fruit and granola it will taste great, but you will have blown through a sizable portion of your daily calorie count. Stay far away from "fruit on the bottom" yogurt lining the shelves at the grocery store. Just reimagine the advertising slogan as "fat on your bottom" to help you avoid enhanced yogurt.

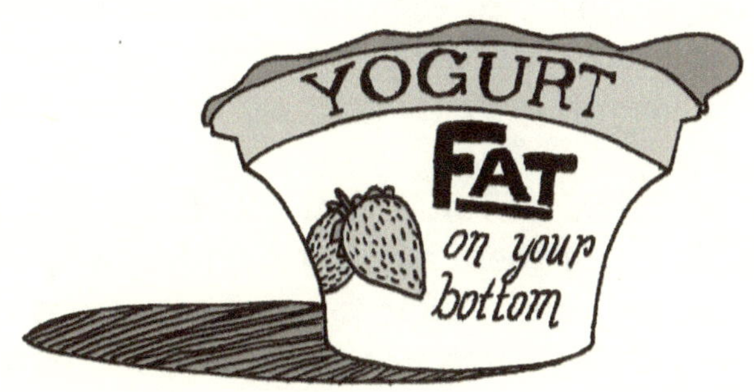

Second, try to avoid eating lunch out. When you are working, try to eat at your desk and go for for a walk. If eating lunch is out is part of the culture at your workplace, make it a once a week treat. My indulgence was "Burger Friday".

At work, beware of the pantry. Nothing good happens in the pan-

try, except the comfortable taste and smell of bad coffee. Your well-meaning and not-so-well-meaning colleagues may often use the pantry as a place to "dump" unwanted calories from home. All sorts of leftover cakes and cookies can magically appear. All for free! Your thoughtful employer may provide you with an endless supply of bagels and donuts, to keep you happy! Stay away. When Henry began corporate employment he quipped that his carb free diet was replaced with a free carb diet...Think about that for a moment and avoid the pantry, except for the burnt coffee.

When you do go a restaurant, pay attention, because everything except the water has calories and you need a plan. Being realistic, you will go over your calorie allotment every time you eat out, so try to limit the damage. Try to avoid the bread basket. A couple of buttered rolls can easily add up to 400 or 500 calories. Beware of salads. Unless they provide a calorie count, assume the calories are high. Cheese, dressing, fruit, nuts, etc. add the calories quickly. Your best choices are usually the grilled meat or fish with vegetables. Skip the bernaise sauce.

Henry here. I echo everything my dad just said, but also wanted to leave you with two things:

First, it isn't realistic to try to always avoid restaurants. Sometimes you will have to eat out. That is life. Plan for it by pre-eating, adjusting your other meals that week, and doing damage control when you are there by ordering something responsible.

Second, be skeptical of fast-casual places that seem relatively healthy. Many of them are, but even those often have huge amounts of sodium in their food, which is not ideal to eat regularly in such high amounts. Some will use fattier cuts of meat than you'd expect to lower their cost - a lot of places offering chicken give you chicken thighs, which have more fat than chicken breasts. With that in mind, there are a lot of good options out there for fast-casual if you are in a pinch, especially those that allow you to make your own customized bowl. This can be helpful, but usually still isn't as good as getting to make the food yourself.

CHAPTER 18: COOKING

◆ ◆ ◆

Unless you happen to have an extravagant amount of money or love spending more than you need to, you are going to need to bite the bullet and cook at least some of your own food. Buying food at restaurants or as takeout is easy, but let's call it what it is: you are paying a group of people to cook something for you, do all the cleanup, and make it tasty. For sit-down spots, add in the waiters coming by every few minutes to check on you and fill up your water, and you realize that a restaurant is a truly luxurious thing. Every employee creating your food needs to get paid.

Thus it shouldn't be surprising that eating out costs a lot more than making food yourself. In my experience, cooking my own meals usually means food is about half the price - or less - of buying it out at takeout places. The price difference is even bigger at more upscale restaurants. Do your wallet a good deed and start cooking most of your meals yourself.

Money aside, cooking your own food is important because you get to pick the ingredients and amounts of them. Everyone knows that a lot of takeout food is delicious because of all the added salt and oil in it, but you may not pay attention to just how much salt and oil you are getting in takeout food. A lot of places, logically, will cut back on the more nutritious ingredients like meat and green vegetables and give you cheaper ones like grains and iceberg lettuce. Depending on your exact desired macros, it can be tough to get enough protein and not overload on either fat or carbs when eating out, simply due to restaurant economics.

Maybe you knew all this already. Hopefully some of the ideas below are new to you and make cooking a bit more manageable.

Buy a pressure cooker. Truly a game-changer. The pressure allows you to tenderize otherwise tough meats and veggies very quickly. You can make any kind of stew in one. You can sauté things like a normal frying pan. Then when you are done, you can put the pot in the fridge with a cover on it and keep munching for days. I have yet to try a recipe where I couldn't just throw a bunch of stuff in the pressure cooker and have it turn out great. Most importantly, it does a decent job of turning chicken breasts into something tender enough where I can have pulled chicken every week, opening up a range of recipes for what is otherwise a terribly bland food.

Cook only once or twice a week. Yes, your leftovers will keep that long. When I first started working, I told myself I was going to cook dinner every night. On the menu: scrambled eggs with cheese, the same every day. Doesn't get much easier than that. Melt butter in pan. Crack eggs in pan. Scramble. Serve. This worked well for a few weeks. Every day I would come home from work, get my pan out, cook the eggs, eat the eggs, wash the pan, and call it a night. Soon I began to dread the whole ritual. Maybe I can just leave the pan in the sink and deal with it tomorrow, I would think to myself. One day, getting home from work around 9, I was so tired I skipped dinner altogether: the mental effort of cooking and washing the pan was too much.

I only made it a few weeks, cooking the simplest of recipes, before the effort overwhelmed me. If you really think you are going to cook a multi-step meal every night, good for you. If you can do that, you either love cooking, or have a lot of time on your hands.

If you want this to be sustainable, you're going to need to

learn to love leftovers or, odds are, you will succumb and will start eating out for time's sake. Cooking for multiple days at once will seem like a lot of work up front, but the magic of not having to clean pots and pans every night will make it worth it.

Not only that, but cooking in a big chunk of time over one or two days gives you something hard to find these days: uninterrupted time. It is a great excuse to spend hours catching up with friends and family on the phone, or to binge watch sports or Netflix.

Pre-portion your meals. This is another small thing, but it adds up. Usually, most people cook their big dish, and then leave it in a big container, scooping out a portion every time they need to eat. Save yourself the mental effort of having to measure and clean out a measuring scoop. Get every serving you are going to eat packaged away before the week even starts, so it becomes grab and go. In addition to saving you time, this helps with portion control. There are a lot of great containers out there - I use stackable plastic BPA-free ones, but also love glass. Glass is heavier and can break, so beware.

Cooking doesn't have to be complicated. You'll find a bunch of fancy recipes with dozens of ingredients out there. If you like that sort of stuff, go crazy. But if not, you can do a lot with a little.

I've spent my entire adult life avoiding opening the 1,100 page Joy of Cooking that my parents gave to me on my 18th birthday, yet I've still managed to cook anywhere from half to 90% of my meals over the past few years. While continuing to worry about how complicated "real cooking" was, I managed to build up a simple repertoire of recipes that get the job done.

I rarely touch recipes with more than 5 ingredients, and base almost all my cooking around salt, pepper, butter, olive oil, and soy sauce. It is hard to mess something up using those. Try making stews and casseroles, which are made to be easy and flexible.

This isn't a recipe book, but a few staples that have been awesome for me:

Lentil Ham Stew: I've subsisted off of this for entire months at a time. Cook your lentils as directed by the packaging. Get frozen peas and carrots and microwave them with a little water and a cover so they steam. Drain the water from the peas and carrots. Cook some chicken thighs (sliced into little bite-sized pieces) in another pan. Throw everything in the lentil pot, especially the grease from the chicken thighs. Add in diced ham and some salt and pepper. Stir and enjoy. If you want a bit more carbs, you can add in potatoes (I slice them and microwave with some water in a covered bowl to soften, then toss in). If you feel like slicing up more veggies, add in onions or garlic. If not, it is delicious on its own, but make sure you add in the ham, which is the most important part for flavor. As far as portions, I would roughly have a pound of dry lentils, two pounds of veggies, and around 3 ounces of ham for every 3 pounds of chicken, but the beauty of this one is that you can change the portions to hit the macros you want.

Crack Chicken: This is the only way I enjoy eating chicken breast. Pressure cook chicken breast and shred it with a fork / spatula. Mix in a bottle of hot sauce, greek yogurt or cream cheese, and a ranch dressing powder packet, stirring until it is all mashed in. This one is very customizable, as the full fat and fat-free cream cheese or yogurt tastes about the same in here, so you can have a delicious way to eat chicken without any fat if you'd like. The portions I use for this are 6 lbs chicken breast, one 5 oz bottle of hot sauce, 1 lb greek yogurt or cream cheese, and 1 packet of ranch. You can also find a million variations online if you Google "Crack Chicken", as it has become a craze.

Oven-roasted veggies: Throw frozen or really any kind of veggies on a baking tray and add salt or any other seasoning you like. Put in oven on 350 degrees until starting to get brown and crispy. Ta-da! They are also decent just pan-fried with oil/butter and soy sauce, but I prefer the roasting as it is easier and the crispy bits are delicious.

Scrambled Eggs: Eggs, salt, pepper, butter. You don't even need cheese if you make these right. Google "Gordon Ramsay eggs" for the formal recipe, but the short version is that you cook them on low heat for a long time and stir them a bunch so they get very fluffy and wonderful. I usually don't even bother with salt anymore and they are still delicious. As mentioned earlier, don't be afraid of adding egg whites here for more protein. The real key here is that scrambled eggs are actually fine as leftovers. As long as you don't overcook them either on the initial cooking or the reheat, they don't lose their texture or flavor. Save yourself from the sadness of boiled eggs and just scramble them.

Chicken Alfredo: Pasta (pick your favorite), chicken thighs, frozen peas, pre-made alfredo sauce (the kind in a glass jar), and if you are feeling fancy, fresh garlic. Cook the chicken in a pan and the pasta in a pot. Microwave the peas in a covered bowl with some water to cook them. Mix it all together and stir. You have to use chicken thighs if you want it to be edible - this tastes like eating paper if you use chicken breasts. Although it seems very decadent, this is actually pretty filling and protein-filled if you do the portions right. I used to make it with 6 lbs chicken thighs, 3 lbs dry pasta, 3 lbs peas, and 2 jars of alfredo, but try playing with the portions. Unlike a lot of the pasta you get at Olive Garden, with these portions, this is a lot more meat and veggies than carbs per serving so isn't as bad for you as it might seem. Keep in mind that the chicken thighs are fatty meat, so you don't need to eat nuts with this to get your fat in.

Steamed and Fried Rice: Rice is the backbone of most of my meals, and is one of the most prevalent grains around the world for a reason. It is cheap and versatile, and on its own, not that caloric. A cup has 45 grams of carbs, 4 grams of protein, and only 200 calories. Concerns about carbs aside, rice on its own isn't going to ruin your physique. I was turned off of rice for a while because every time I made it, it got super sticky and was a pain to eat. That comes from overcooking it, which causes it to swell up with extra water and get sticky. You can avoid that by turning the heat off as soon as your timer is up, when there is still a tiny bit of water left in the pot, or getting a rice-cooker that does it for you.

The magic of rice really comes after you've cooked it and had it in your fridge for a day, which makes it better for frying. Throw some in a pan, add any veggies or meat you want, add some soy sauce, any other seasoning you'd like, maybe crack an egg in there, and mix it good, and bam - you've got tasty fried rice. There's a reason fried rice is a staple in many cultures: it is the ultimate leftover dish and you can throw almost anything in it and have a delicious outcome.

A final suggestion on cooking: try making your own desserts. When I usually have dessert, I have a vague idea that it is packed with sugar, but that thought dies the second I have my first bite and go to dessert Valhalla. Things hit a lot closer to home when I have to make it myself and see the shovel-fulls of sugar going in. Not only will doing a bit of the work likely slow you down enough to make you question if it is worth it, you also have to acknowledge that it is a sugar-fest, which might give you a bit more perspective at a restaurant when ordering.

One dessert recipe I've gotten a lot of mileage out of is fried apples. A smidge of butter and some sliced apples in a pan, fried until browned, and doused in cinnamon, tastes delicious and is much healthier than most desserts.

Mark here - I know that Henry provided a number of recipes. I want to add just one. I cook a number of variations on this meal. It is easy, cheap, healthy, low calorie, and very satiating. I like to make a large batch of 8 servings so I can avoiding cooking for a few days and put some away in the freezer. It started out as a version of a French Cassoulet. Think of it as French Chili!

2 pounds meat. I usually use a mix of low fat ground pork and ground chicken. You can used sliced chicken breast and sliced pork if you prefer. Just about any meat will do, but keep it lean. I never use beef as it has more fat than the dish needs.

1.5 cups of dried beans soaked overnight and rinsed

1 pound chopped carrots (I use frozen versions of the carrots, cauliflower, and green beans to minimize effort)

1 pound (head) of cauliflower

1 pound cut green beans

24 ounces of chopped tomatoes (I use a boxed brand, but cans are also fine)

1 tablespoon each of black pepper, minced onion, garlic powder

2 tablespoons of oregano

1 teaspoon each of salt and fennel seed Small amount of red pepper flakes

The easiest way to cook this is in a pressure cooker.

Sauté the meat in olive oil

Add all other ingredients, stir

Cook on chili setting for 35 minutes, vent.

Separately, if you want to cook it in a Dutch oven, the steps are the same as above but simmer on the stove top for several hours with a lid slightly off or in the oven for several hours at 275.

Now go out there and save money and calories by cooking your own meals!

CHAPTER 19: HOW EXERCISE FITS INTO IT

◆ ◆ ◆

You probably think I'm an idiot for having a chapter on walking and another chapter on exercise, because walking is a form of exercise.

Technically, you are right, it is. But thinking about walking as exercise is wrong. Walking is life.

Walking is what gets us from point A to point B. Without walking, we are forced into wheelchairs or to crawl like babies. Walking is a given unless you are grossly unhealthy. But once you get to the point where walking is as easy as breathing, you may want to up the ante a little bit.

Earlier in the book, I hinted about how running burns more calories than walking, but was a bit negative on running in general. That is because I think that exercise has a far more noble purpose than simply being a vehicle to burn calories.

Let's use an investing metaphor. You have two options:

Option 1: You work for every dollar you spend. You stuff any extra money you make under your mattress.

Option 2: You invest your extra money. At first, it seems like small peanuts, but over the years, the size of your account grows, and the magic of compound interest takes effect. Decades later, a large portion of your spending can be funded by your investments. You don't have to work nearly as hard and you cut back your work hours to spend more time enjoying your life.

Which option sounds better to you? Option one means you get out exactly what you put in. Option two gives you more than that. Option one is the equivalent to exercising just to burn calories, and option two is the equivalent to adding in strength training to build muscle. This is why you should be doing strength training to build muscle instead of only doing cardiovascular activity like walking, running or biking.

Fat does not burn calories. Your body burns fat for energy to power its activities. Your brain needs a lot of energy. So does your heart, and your liver, and your other organs. So do your muscles. The bigger and more active your brain is, the more energy you'll burn. Sadly, you can't make your organs any larger. You can make your heart work harder through cardio, but that is more like option one. Your muscles, however, can be trained to grow larger. The larger they are, the more calories they burn. This is the part of your metabolism you may have the most control over.

I hear people complain all the time about how their metabolism has slowed down as they got older. Yes, some of that happened naturally, but a lot was likely because they stopped exercising and getting stronger like they used to. They lost muscle mass and now their metabolism has dropped because they have less muscle around to burn calories, and sadly, they just can't eat as much as they used to without gaining weight.

Nobody can seem to agree on how many calories a pound of muscle burns. People used to say that a pound of muscle burns an extra fifty calories per day. That number has now been backed down to around five calories per day[40], and will continue to be studied. Not only that, but muscle is much denser than fat, so a pound of muscle is much smaller. Two individuals the same weight, one with more muscle than the other, will find that the more muscular one is actually smaller.

Think of your muscles like engines that need a lot of fuel. The bigger they get, the more fuel they burn even when idling. This is the interest you are earning on them. Even more importantly, when you fire them up, and challenge them to lift heavy objects or work hard, they burn a lot of calories.

The stronger you are, the more calories you burn from every workout because you have more muscle mass firing. At the end of the day, it is a physics equation. You need more energy to move more mass. Therefore, the more muscle you can put on, the more calories you will burn both sitting and during your workouts.

The snowball effect continues when we return to the tables about walking. Heavier individuals burn more calories when they walk. Muscle is heavy. If you can gain more muscle, your walks become even more effective and becoming lean becomes even easier.

Strangely, trying to build more muscle is almost like a lazy-man's approach to getting lean. You could run for hours each day, convincing your body to lose all muscle not required for running, but as you do this, your metabolism will drop as you get lighter and have less muscle mass. You'll have to run for longer to burn the same amount of calories.

Or, you could strength train and build more muscle. The more muscle you build, the more calories you will burn with the same amount of exercise. One is a vicious cycle, one is a virtuous one. This vicious cycle of cardio only is why sometimes you see people who are "cardio bunnies" that only run on the treadmill, and despite running inhuman distances regularly, are still somewhat doughey. They get even more frustrated and eat even less, spiraling further, Sometimes this leads to anorexia. Good outcomes become tougher and tougher to reach.

The wonderful thing about focusing on muscle is that it is health-inducing. You can judge your muscle health and strength by its performance, by how much weight it can move. If your performance starts to drop, you know you need to rest or eat more. To maintain a constant level of strength, you can't just starve yourself. With running or cardio, you can sometimes fudge things by just grinding on and pushing harder. For endurance activities, that may work, but when you are trying to lift hundreds of pounds, a bit more grit just won't cut it - you need muscle power, not just willpower. Therefore, if someone uses their strength as a barometer, rather than endurance, they are less likely to starve themself into an unhealthy body state.

You Can't Out-Train a Bad Diet

The fattest and heaviest I've been since high school was during my summer internship after my junior year of college. It was also when I was working out the most I have since high school. I would wake up and immediately do a circuit of three supersets of bodyweight exercises - pushups, squats, handstand pushups, pull-ups, and leg raises - two per day, rotating every day. Then, I would get dressed and go to the gym to lift for an hour. Then after work, I would either lift for another hour or rock climb for two.

That summer, I had decided that it was time to bulk up. I was going to gain some muscle mass, and accepted that some fat would come with it. I was eating an unbelievable amount of food, and was painfully full every day that summer. It worked. I was ecstatic with my weight gain, and felt like I still had my abs. Everything was going better than I could have hoped. My shirts were getting tight. I felt huge.

In late July, I went on a road trip with a few buddies that ended up with us swimming in a lake, and a friend commenting on my "gut". This was my "know thy belly" moment that summer. It hurt, but I still couldn't really see it myself and decided to cut weight because I trusted my buddies. It was only later when I cut down, taking progress pictures as I leaned out, that I was able to see that I had packed on some extra lard. Most importantly, I learned that even training as much as I was, that still didn't mean I would stay lean.

If you are going to eat crappy foods, know that unless you are exercising most of the day, your body composition is probably going to suffer. Not only that, but you are doing things the hard way: you are eating garbage and then having to exercise more to compensate. Wouldn't it be more productive to just eat healthy so you can spend that time doing something enriching to your life, instead of just mindlessly trying to burn calories?

Even if you are eating healthy foods, if you are eating too much food, you will gain weight, and often, that weight will include some fat with it. Even if you are exercising a lot, if you eat too much, you will still likely get fatter.

Pour Some Sugar on Me

While you will likely fail if you try to out-exercise a bad diet, exercise will mitigate the effects of the bad foods you do eat to some extent. This means that if you are dead set on eating sugar and high glycemic carbohydrates, the best time to do it is right after or during a tough workout.

In fact, some athletes and bodybuilders are actually encouraged to load up on quickly digesting carbs (sugar) and protein during and after their workouts. That is part of the marketing pitch of sports drinks. This sounded like heresy when I first read it. I had been led to believe that sugar is the root of all evil. How was it that professional athletes, who in theory, had access to the best sports nutritionists that money could buy, be so stupid as to eat pure sugar willingly?

Eventually I came to discover that sugar in general is bad, but when you are exercising, the playing field shifts. When straining your muscles during high intensity activity involving power movements such as in weight lifting, you are quickly burning energy stores. If you want to replenish those stores in a manner that allows you to maintain your performance during that workout, pure sugar is the fastest way to do that. Similarly, right after a workout, your muscles are desperate for energy and protein, so a shake with quick-digesting sugar and whey protein is the best way to replenish them.

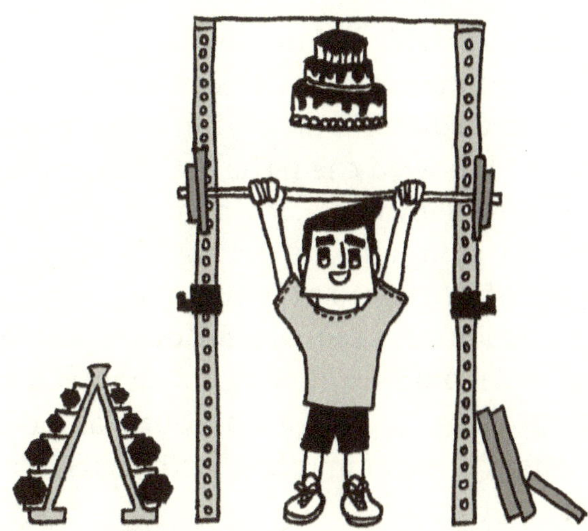

I refused to believe this until I was able to run a little experiment on myself to test my own blood sugar levels and how they were affected by a sugary drink during a workout.

A good friend of mine has type I diabetes, an auto-immune disorder in which the body is unable to produce its own insulin. To survive, he must monitor his blood sugar level and give himself man-made insulin to keep his blood sugar in a healthy range.

There are a few ways that diabetics do this. He prefers the lower-tech way: using a finger prick test. Every few hours, he pricks his finger and places a drop of blood onto a disposable plastic strip which is inserted into a monitor that reads his blood sugar level. If it is too low, he has to eat carbs. If it is too high, he has to inject insulin. He has to be acutely aware of his blood sugar at all times because unlike most people, his body will not regulate it on its own.

However, he also has a higher tech version, a continuous glucose monitor ("CGM") called Dexcom. This is a device straight out of the Matrix. You insert a needle into your stomach, tape a patch over it, and have a little pager device that tells you your blood sugar levels every five minutes, charting it on a line graph so you can watch the levels change over time. Every few hours you have to calibrate the Dexcom by pricking your finger and testing it with the old-fashioned monitor.

He allowed me to experiment with this kit in college. While a lot of using it just resulted in me trying to get people to gasp in the library when I showed them the patch on my stomach or pricked out blood from my finger, it was most instructive when I brought it into the gym with me during a heavy leg workout. This was the kind of workout I only had the time and stamina to do in college: two hours of squats, deadlifts, and leg presses. During my session, I would sip a sports drink mixed with whey protein to test out if sugar during a workout was indeed beneficial. The blood sugar test was my chance to see if it was actually doing anything.

I watched my blood sugar levels the whole workout and didn't drink any at first to see if my blood sugar would plunge without it. As expected, my blood sugar dropped throughout the workout, getting well below 100 maybe 30 minutes into the heavy lifting. That meant it was abnormally low, which made sense, as I was dizzy and exhausted. I chugged a huge swig of sports drink and carried on. In the next blood sugar reading, I could see my blood sugar come back up to normal levels.

I kept drinking the sports drink and whey combo and was able to keep my blood sugar normal throughout the workout because of it. I tried this again over the next few days, with the same result: during my heavy workouts, my blood sugar would drop, and the sports drink would bring it up to normal levels. It was amazing to see, firsthand, sugar's ability to regulate my blood sugar levels during exercise, disbanding my original notion of sugar having zero positive attributes.

I share this story not to encourage everyone to drink whey and sports drinks during workouts. Some people may not respond well. If you are seriously overweight, you may have elevated blood sugar and not need any more. Do some more research on it before deciding it is right for you. However, I share the story to make two main points:

Don't be dogmatic. Just because you read something and

everyone has decided it is true doesn't mean it is. I was convinced that sugar was terrible, and then I found this loophole. Nutrition and the human body is a very complicated topic that is always changing. Know that what is "true" today may not be true in a decade. Keep testing, keep learning, keep challenging, and be ready to be proven wrong.

There are ways to do damage control. If you've decided you can't live without sugar, eat it after your workout. It will help. If you are interested in this, Tim Ferriss wrote in depth about practices and supplements that you can use to eat lots of food without gaining weight in his book *The Four Hour Body*.

Where to Start

Hopefully by now you are pumped up about adding some strength training to your life and putting on some muscle mass to get your metabolism revved up. If so, you're probably rearing to go.

This isn't a book on weightlifting so I will keep the recommendations light, but will say one thing: if you don't have experience with strength training, you can get a lot of mileage out of simple bodyweight training. I'm talking old school push-ups, pull-ups, bodyweight squats, bridges, leg raises, and handstands and handstand pushups. You don't necessarily have to go to a gym right away, especially if you still have a good amount of weight to lose. Your body is probably more than heavy enough for you to make progress using just these exercises. There are a lot of great progressions on body weight exercises, so start there while you research what lifting program to do.

When you decide to start lifting weights, I would highly recommend that you find a trainer or strength coach to help teach you the proper form before you just go start squatting, deadlifting, or bench pressing on your own. You can learn a lot of it on the internet, but nothing can replace having someone actually coach your form live.

The world of lifting is infinitely complicated, with dozens of different approaches to how many sets and reps to do, which exercises are best, how long to rest between sets, how many days to train per week, and how often you should take de-load weeks to recover. Dozens of books have been written on the subject, but broadly you should rest easy knowing that many people have had a lot of success with different approaches, so there is not a right one for everyone.

Sometimes, an approach that used to work for you will stop working. Exercises you used to love may now hurt your joints. Try new ones and find the ones that work best for you. You may find that you are no longer making progress, which may call for changing your rep scheme, using lighter weights, or using heavier weights. There are a lot of possible solutions, and I suggest spending more time reading or talking to a trainer or coach to learn more.

Most importantly, as you get into muscle-building training, know it can help you burn calories, and can help you build muscle to increase your metabolism. However, as mentioned, if you are eating too much and eating the wrong things, exercise will not magically transform your physique. There are plenty of lifters that are very strong but also very fat - muscle does not automatically make you lean. You still have to pay attention to your diet. For this reason, I have included exercise last in the order of things you need to do for results.

Good luck, and happy strength training!

Mark here - Henry has given a tremendous amount of good information on exercise, so I will keep it brief. In my 50's, I try to keep relatively fit without injuring myself. Everyday I get 30 minutes of exercise through fast walking, at least 5 miles or 10,000 steps or five miles of total walking, and I work out with free weights every other day. Beyond that I'm active at home and in my hobbies. Just enough, without getting hurt.

As I've gotten older I've discovered that when lifting weights, lighter weights + more reps is a great way to avoid joint injuries.

Beyond the maintenance exercise I described above, you can change your body composition if you are motivated enough, I'll defer to the exercise professionals on the how to's.

CHAPTER 20: YOU DID IT. NOW WHAT?

◆ ◆ ◆

We've completed our normal curriculum.

Sure, there are more layers: the rabbit hole goes as deep as you want it to. Doctors and nutritionists will continue to make breakthroughs every year. But you have the tools you need. Everything else is just icing.

Now you have to do the hardest part: execute.

Maybe you already have executed and currently have the body you've always wanted. If so, nice work, but it doesn't stop now. Remember the octopus? It never dies and never gives up, no matter how much progress you've made. It will always try to rope you back in when it gets a chance.

Life will always pose challenges for you. Weddings, parties, emergencies, children, business trips, mid-life crises. "Unknown unknowns" will appear and throw obstacles at your dieting progress. The key is having a plan in place to work around them, rather than short-circuiting and lamenting your perfect routine being messed up. Life happens, and unless you choose to live in a bubble, things will always come up that complicate your diet, so you need to have a strong framework to adapt.

We have already built most of this framework throughout the book:

Make it Small and Sustainable: Consider the sustainability of any diet you start before starting it.

Know Thy Belly: Be aware of what your weight is and what it should be.

Tool Box: Track your progress so you know how changes affect your body.

Start with Soda: Start by cutting sugary drinks. If you avoid them, you dodge a major landmine.

Sleep Yourself Skinny: Make sure you get enough sleep when you can, so you don't weaken your willpower and mess up your hormones to make you hungrier.

One Step at a Time: Build regular walks into your routine to create a recurring calorie-burning activity.

Live, Fast, and Die Old: See how your body responds to intermittent fasting. It will teach you to be more in tune with your hunger. Avoid snacks. Make sure if you eat, you are having something with nutritional value.

The Fat and Happy Scale: Take it all gradually and be mindful of the fact that your body will try to stop you if you change things too fast. Plan for your progress to be lumpy, not linear.

What to Eat / Navigating the Food Spectrum: Focus your diet around lean meats, veggies, and complex carbohydrates.
How Much to Eat: Be mindful of portion sizes and change them to achieve your goals.

Required vs Extracurricular Eating: Eat healthy foods every day before you eat unhealthy ones, and be flexible if you need to.

Cooking: Cook your own foods and don't keep junk food

around.

How Exercise Fits Into It: Try exercising to build muscle and increase your metabolism.

Now, the final piece of the puzzle is planning your weight for the long term. Obviously, you want to maintain the habits above, in addition to any other beneficial ones you have discovered yourself. But this is a battle and you need more than that.

Since the unknown unknowns and the octopus can sneak up on you at any moment, you need to be ready for bad things to happen. To do that, once you find your target weight, plan to spend most of your time about two pounds below it. That way, if suddenly someone robs you and says:

"Give me your wallet, and eat this whole box of donuts or I'll kill you!"

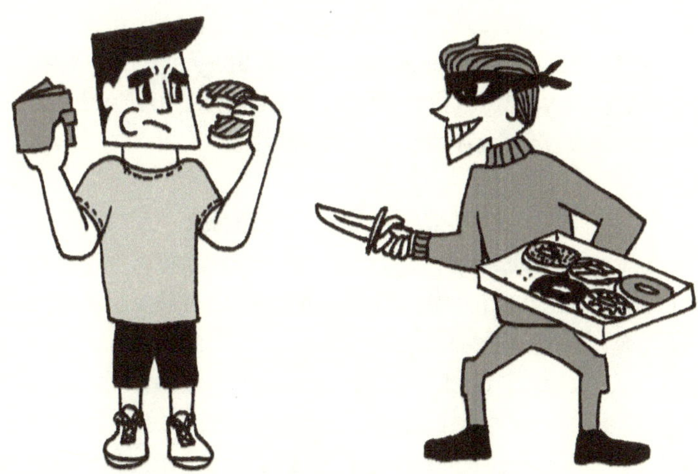

After this odd food-pushing criminal steals all your money, you will at least have one thing to smile about: your physique isn't ruined. You gain two pounds, and suddenly you will be at your target weight anyway. This way, you have a buffer zone for any shenanigans that enter your life. You don't have to feel guilty for breaking your diet. This way, when someone wants to go out for burgers or pizza, you can do it and not worry.

In addition to living a little bit below your target weight, you should accept the fact that you are going to get older and that it will affect your body.

As you age, your muscles will shrink and your metabolism will decline. You will have to eat less calories to maintain the same weight. Just because you don't like it doesn't make it any less true. Therefore, accept the fact that next year you may have to eat less than you do this year. Your weight and physique should drive your outcomes, not a set amount of calories you want to eat or think you should eat. You have to react to reality, not your desires.

The inevitable fact of aging is why I am such a strong advocate for strength training. At a certain age, any muscle you have will start to atrophy, so the more you can build until then, the longer you will have not only a stronger body, but also a higher metabolism.

So, the only constant is change and that annoying octopus trying to get you to sabotage yourself. Stay strong, stay consistent, and plan for yourself to slip sometimes. Just get ready to get back up and keep fighting the good fight.

You are the Scientist

As you continue on your fitness journey, there's a good chance that at some point, after implementing the ideas in this book, you will want to deepen your understanding of why these concepts work and test variations of them. This means the training wheels are coming off, and you are looking to tweak the diet to work better for you. This is you taking ownership for seeing how things work for your body.

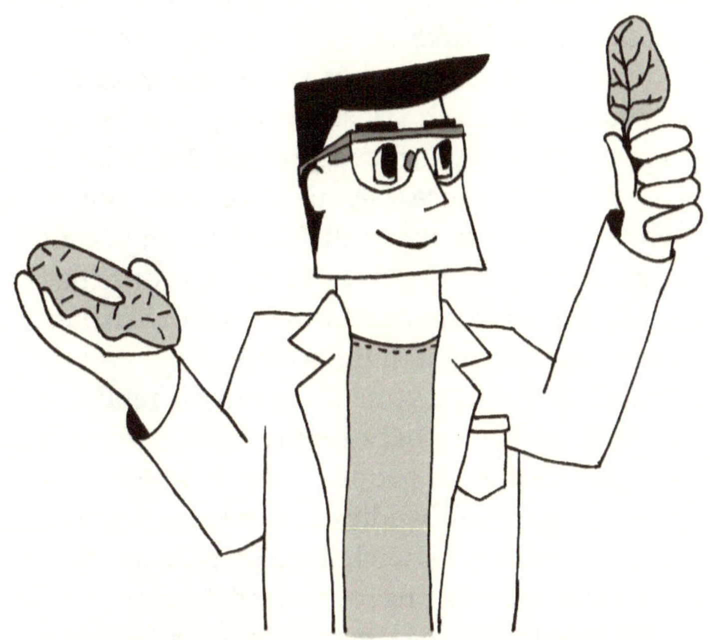

As you do this, you may look towards academic studies on fitness and nutrition. These are a good start, and they will give you directional guidance, but not everything you find in studies will work on you, and not all studies are things you can replicate in your own life. Your circumstances are unique. Your weight, your athletic history, your emotional habits, your commute, and your social circle are uniquely yours, and may skew any studies you try on yourself to give you different results than you read about.

This doesn't mean the science isn't valid. Some studies capture a response to a change in variable only for a limited population. A study on elderly women may not apply to young men, but it also may. It isn't always clear. If it doesn't apply to you, that doesn't mean the study is wrong, but that your body is different from the test subjects'. It may not apply to you now, but years later it also might. You can't be certain.

There is really only one way to find out: test it for yourself and take ownership for the results. If the science isn't applicable to you, do your own science and seek the truth for yourself.

Not even all scientists and industry experts agree on everything, so you shouldn't take everything as truth. Find what works for you and go with that, but know that your body will change and you may need to try something new later in your life. There are nuggets of truth everywhere. Don't be afraid to learn about them just because they disagree with your view.

This is why there are so many different diets: because they all work to an extent. You just have to find the one that works best for you, and before you even do that, start with basics that supersede the nuances of an individual diet.

Keep in mind that while your attempts to replicate some studies will result in failure because the studies were only applicable to narrow ranges of people, some studies and articles pretending to be legitimate studies are actually just total crap. A lot of times this happens with studies that are funded by companies or industries that have a vested interest in a certain outcome. This happens all the time. Dig a little deeper into the background of a study if you have time and see who is paying for it, and who is doing it.

Easier to see through, however, is advertisements or testimonials for supplements or diets done by celebrities or pro athletes that suggest their success is due to that supplement or diet. The celebrities are not famous because of the cucumber face mask they are using, they are advertising the cucumber face mask because they are famous. The athletes that endorse some shiny pre-workout powder and claim it is the key to their gains are getting paid to say that.

Sometimes there is truth behind these testimonials, but not always. Be skeptical, and before you shell out a bunch of money for some miracle supplement, look for published studies on its efficacy. See if there are multiple studies or just one that was published right when the product got published. Look for meta-studies that incorporate dozens of other studies to draw more definitive conclusions. More importantly, remember that supplements are meant to be supplemental, not the mainstay of your health program. Get the big things right, and then tinker with supplements if you still find it necessary.

Dieting for Decades

These are the basics. If you can do these, and continue doing them, you don't need to become a registered dietician. You don't need a bunch of fancy supplements. You don't need crazy genetics. You just need to be consistent and have a system. Once you get in your groove, stay in it. If you want to go to the next level of precision and go into the weeds on these things, have fun. There's plenty out there to learn, and the nuances of the field are always changing. But whatever you do, don't lose sight of the forest amidst the trees. If you are getting these basic principles wrong, all the fancy science and methods in the world won't help you.

There is no magic. Just focus, planning, persistency, and continuous learning. You don't need any miracle food or supplement. If you continue to follow these principles, things will work out, and you can stop stressing about your diet so much, and do what you really wanted to do in the first place: go live your life and focus on more important things.

ACKNOWLEDGE-MENTS

◆ ◆ ◆

For a book that I tried to keep secret from almost everyone I know while I wrote it, this got a lot of love from those close to me.

Dad, thank you for co-writing, even though I know you don't enjoy it nearly as much as I did. Without your perspective, this book would be half-baked and not nearly as relevant for many people.

Mom, you encouraged me from day one, and have always challenged me to push myself while not coming off as overbearing. That is a rare gift. Thank you for everything, including humoring me on all my strange food requests over the years. Thank you for reading all the drafts and helping me tighten my focus.

To my incredible sister Rachel, thank you for being a sounding board on ideas, and for your early read of the book. You also took a killer author photo - thank you for your photography skills.

Dan R, Dan H, Paul G, Kyle H, and Jack H, thank you for your close reads and insightful edits. You helped refine and shape this book into what it is today. I'm lucky to call you guys my friends.

Missy Quick, thank you for giving this book a beautiful set of illustrations, and for helping brainstorm ways to improve my initial set of ideas.

Shelby T, Sarah P, and Brittany S, thank you for sharing your insights into publishing. Your insight was greatly helpful in understanding how to turn this from an idea to a book.

Morgan M, the book you got me for Christmas in 2018 was part of my inspiration to actually finally write this. Thank you for that, and thank you for your patience and support as I locked myself away on weekends to write.

Covercreators (Pradeep) on Fiverr, thank you for building an awesome cover.

The folks at Renaissance Periodization, thank you for helping me deepen my knowledge of nutrition, and for allowing me to use one of your images in the book.

All the other fitness and nutrition authors and coaches who have helped me over the years, thank you.

Everyone else who has had to hear me talk about this project as I've worked on it, thank you. I appreciate your support and encouragement.

ABOUT THE AUTHORS

◆ ◆ ◆

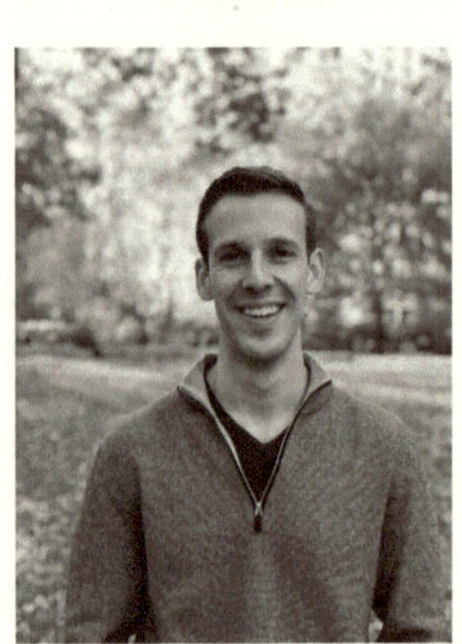

Henry Barry is currently an employee in the asset management industry, residing in New York City. After spending most of his childhood in Singapore as the son of an ex-pat and living in seven states in the US, he loves seeing new places and trying new food. Henry is passionate about helping create efficient systems for people to achieve goals in their lives, whether health-related or otherwise. In his spare time, he enjoys reading, rock climbing, weight lifting, and spending time with friends. Henry holds the Chartered Financial Analyst designation (CFA Institute ID: 8305170) and is a proud graduate of Washington University in St. Louis, with a major in Economics and a minor in Writing.

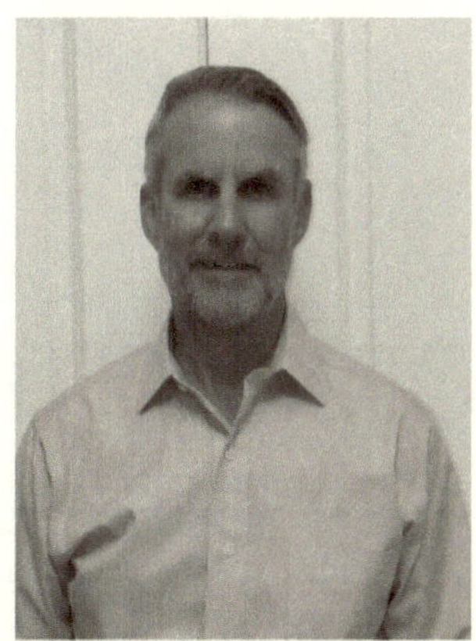

Mark Barry worked for more than three decades in corporate roles serving as division president for four different companies. He lived and worked internationally for many years and developed an appreciation for different cultures and perspectives. Today he is an independent company board member and performs consulting work in private equity. Mark believes that nutrition and fitness are key to well being and longevity. He resides in Florida and is passionate about boating with his wife and friends.

WORKS CITED

[1] "Overweight & Obesity Statistics." *National Institute of Diabetes and Digestive and Kidney Diseases*, U.S. Department of Health and Human Services, 1 Aug. 2017, www.niddk.nih.gov/health-information/health-statistics/overweight-obesity.

[2] "Report on the Economic Well-Being of U.S. Households in 2017." *Board of Governors of the Federal Reserve System*, May 2018, www.federalreserve.gov/publications/report-economic-well-being-us-households.htm.

[3] "Sightlines Financial Security Special Report: Seeing Our Way to Financial Security in the Age of Increased Longevity." *Longevity.stanford.edu*, Oct. 2018, longevity.stanford.edu/sightlines-financial-security-special-report-mobile/.

[4] "Calories Burned by Occupation." *CalorieLab Calorie Counter*, calorielab.com/burned/?mo=se&gr=11&ti=Occupation&wt=150&un=lb&kg=68.

[5] Curry, Andrew. "The Gladiator Diet." *Archaeology Magazine Archive*, 2008, archive.archaeology.org/0811/abstracts/gladiator.html.

[6] Martinez, Keilah E, et al. "Expanded Normal Weight Obesity and Insulin Resistance in US Adults of the National Health and Nutrition Examination Survey." *Journal of Diabetes Research*, Hindawi, 25 July 2017, www.hindawi.com/journals/jdr/2017/9502643/.

[7] UHN Staff. "Symptoms of Reactive Hypoglycemia and Insulin Resistance." *University Health News*, 30 Nov. 2018, universityhealthnews.com/daily/diabetes/feeling-sleepy-all-the-time-and-chronic-fatigue-are-reactive-hypoglycemia-and-

insulin-resistance-symptoms/.

[8] "Osteoarthritis : Role of Body Weight in Osteoarthritis - Weight Management." *Johns Hopkins Arthritis Center*, www.hopkinsarthritis.org/patient-corner/disease-management/role-of-body-weight-in-osteoarthritis/#joint.

[9] "FastStats - Overweight Prevalence." *Centers for Disease Control and Prevention*, Centers for Disease Control and Prevention, 13 June 2016, www.cdc.gov/nchs/fastats/obesity-overweight.htm.

[10] Harvard Health Publishing. "Ask the Doctor: Do Artificial Sweeteners Cause Insulin Resistance?" *Harvard Health*, Feb. 2017, www.health.harvard.edu/diabetes/ask-the-doctor-do-artificial-sweeteners-cause-insulin-resistance.

[11] Williamson, A, and A Feyer. "Moderate Sleep Deprivation Produces Impairments in Cognitive and Motor Performance Equivalent to Legally Prescribed Levels of Alcohol Intoxication." *Occupational and Environmental Medicine*, BMJ Group, Oct. 2000, www.ncbi.nlm.nih.gov/pmc/articles/PMC1739867/.

[12] Greer, Stephanie M, et al. "The Impact of Sleep Deprivation on Food Desire in the Human Brain." *Nature Communications*, U.S. National Library of Medicine, 2013, www.ncbi.nlm.nih.gov/pmc/articles/PMC3763921/.

[13] Easton, John. "New Study Helps Explain Links between Sleep Loss and Diabetes." *Science Life*, University of Chicago Medicine, 19 Feb. 2015, sciencelife.uchospitals.edu/2015/02/19/new-study-helps-explain-links-between-sleep-loss-and-diabetes/.

[14] Leproult, Rachel, and Eve Van Cauter. "Role of Sleep and Sleep Loss in Hormonal Release and Metabolism." *Endocrine Development*, U.S. National Library of Medicine, 2010, www.ncbi.nlm.nih.gov/pmc/articles/PMC3065172/.

[15] Beccuti, Guglielmo, and Silvana Pannain. "Sleep and Obesity." *Current Opinion in Clinical Nutrition and Metabolic Care*, U.S. National Library of Medicine, July 2011, www.ncbi.nlm.nih.gov/pmc/articles/PMC3632337/.

[16] "Melatonin and Sleep." *National Sleep Foundation*, www.sleepfoundation.org/articles/melatonin-and-sleep.

[17] "Melatonin Dosage: Sleep.org by the National Sleep Foundation." *Sleep.org*, www.sleep.org/articles/how-much-melatonin-to-take/.

[18] https://justgetflux.com/

[19] "Home." *Calories Burned HQ*, caloriesburnedhq.com/.

[20] Mayo Clinic Staff. "The Best Ways to Cut Calories from Your Diet." *Mayo Clinic*, Mayo Foundation for Medical Education and Research, 28 Mar. 2018, www.mayoclinic.org/healthy-lifestyle/weight-loss/in-depth/calories/art-20048065.

[21] Hijikata, Yasuyo, and Seika Yamada. "Walking Just after a Meal Seems to Be More Effective for Weight Loss than Waiting for One Hour to Walk after a Meal." *International Journal of General Medicine*, Dove Medical Press, 2011, www.ncbi.nlm.nih.gov/pmc/articles/PMC3119587/.

[22] Wong, May. "Stanford Study Finds Walking Improves Creativity." *Stanford News*, 24 Apr. 2014, news.stanford.edu/2014/04/24/walking-vs-sitting-042414/.

[23] Dean, Nicole. "Stepping Up Your Creativity: Walking, Meditation, and the Creative Brain " Brain World." *Brain World*, 29 Mar. 2019, brainworldmagazine.com/stepping-creativity-walking-meditation-creative-brain/.

[24] Tello, Monique. "Intermittent Fasting: Surprising Update." *Harvard Health Blog*, 26 June 2018, www.health.harvard.edu/blog/intermittent-fasting-surprising-update-2018062914156.

[25] "Intermittent Fasting: No Advantage over Conventional Weight Loss Diets." *ScienceDaily*, ScienceDaily, 26 Nov. 2018, www.sciencedaily.com/releases/2018/11/181126115842.htm.

[26] "Menstruation: Missed Periods in Athletes (Athletic Amenorrhea)." *Summit Medical Group*, 2014, www.summitmedicalgroup.com/library/adult_health/sma_athletic_amenorrhea/.

[27] Hathaway, Bill. "Sugar Targets Gut Microbe Linked to Lean and Healthy People." *YaleNews*, 17 Dec. 2018, news.yale.edu/2018/12/17/sugar-targets-gut-microbe-

linked-lean-and-healthy-people.

[28] Nutrition Data - Know What You Eat, nutritiondata.self.com/.

[29] Clayton, Paul. "How to Incorporate Lean Meats Into Your Diet." *MeatScience.org*, 31 May 2017, meatscience.org/ TheMeatWeEat/topics/fresh-meat/article/2017/05/31/how-to-incorporate-lean-meats-in-your-diet.

[30] "Glycogen: An Overview." *ScienceDirect*, www.sciencedirect.com/topics/neuroscience/glycogen.

[31] LeWine, Howard. "Fish Oil: Friend or Foe?" *Harvard Health Blog*, Harvard Medical School, 24 July 2019, www.health.harvard.edu/blog/fish-oil-friend-or-foe-201307126467.

[32] Center for Food Safety and Applied Nutrition. "Mercury Levels in Commercial Fish and Shellfish (1990-2012)." *U.S. Food and Drug Administration*, FDA, 25 Oct. 2017, www.fda.gov/food/ metals/mercury-levels-commercial-fish-and-shellfish-1990-2012.

[33] Seymour, Tom. "Are Organ Meats Good for You?" *Medical News Today*, MediLexicon International, 3 Sept. 2017, www.medicalnewstoday.com/articles/319229.php.

[34] "Eggs Might Help Your Heart, Not Harm It." *Harvard Health*, Harvard Medical School, Aug. 2018, www.health.harvard.edu/ heart-health/eggs-might-help-your-heart-not-harm-it.

[35] Hong-Brown, L Q, et al. "Alcohol Impairs Protein Synthesis and Degradation in Cultured Skeletal Muscle Cells." *Alcoholism, Clinical and Experimental Research*, U.S. National Library of Medicine, Sept. 2001, www.ncbi.nlm.nih.gov/pubmed/11584159.

[36] "How Alcohol Affects the Quality-And Quantity-Of Sleep." *National Sleep Foundation*, www.sleepfoundation.org/articles/ how-alcohol-affects-quality-and-quantity-sleep.

[37] "The Truth about Fats: the Good, the Bad, and the in-Between." *Harvard Health*, Harvard Medical School, 13 Aug. 2018, www.health.harvard.edu/staying-healthy/the-truth-about-fats-bad-and-good.

[38] Hurst, Yumi, and Haruhisa Fukuda. "Effects of Changes in

Eating Speed on Obesity in Patients with Diabetes: a Secondary Analysis of Longitudinal Health Check-up Data." *BMJ Open*, BMJ Publishing Group, 12 Feb. 2018, www.ncbi.nlm.nih.gov/pubmed/29440054.

[39] Angelopoulos, Theodoros, et al. "The Effect of Slow Spaced Eating on Hunger and Satiety in Overweight and Obese Patients with Type 2 Diabetes Mellitus." *BMJ Open Diabetes Research & Care*, BMJ Publishing Group, 2 July 2014, www.ncbi.nlm.nih.gov/pmc/articles/PMC4212566/.

[40] "A Pound of Muscle Burns 30-50 Kcal/Day, Really…." *National Council on Strength & Fitness*, www.ncsf.org/enew/articles/articles-poundofmuscle.aspx.